CELIAC DISEASE COOKBOOK FOR BEGINNERS

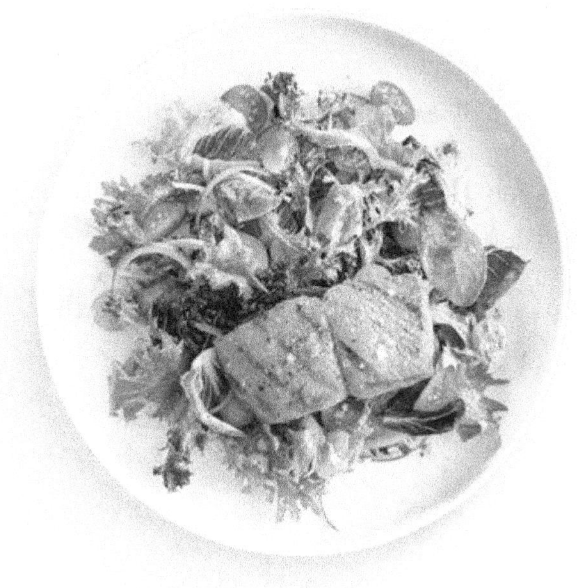

Gluten-Free Tempting and Flavorful Recipes for Starters to Savor Every Bite and Boost Healthy Wellbeing

Joan G. Milone

Copyright © 2024 by Joan G. Milone

All rights reserved.

No part of this book may be reproduced, stored in a retrieval system, or transmitted in any form or by any means, electronic, mechanical, photocopying, recording, or otherwise, without prior written permission of the copyright owner.

This book is written as a source of information only. The information contained in this book is provided in good faith and is believed to be accurate and reliable as of the date of publication. The author does not assume any responsibility for any errors or omissions that may appear.

FIVE EASY STEPS TO MAKE THE MOST OUT OF THIS COOKBOOK:

1. Start by familiarizing yourself with the cookbook's layout and organization. Flip through the pages to get a sense of the recipes, ingredients, and cooking techniques involved.

2. Take note of the recipe index and table of contents. Identify recipes that appeal to you and align with your dietary preferences and restrictions related to celiac disease.

3. Begin with simple recipes that require minimal ingredients and cooking steps. Gradually build confidence in your gluten-free cooking skills before attempting more complex dishes.

4. Gather all necessary ingredients and equipment before starting a recipe. Double-check labels to ensure they are gluten-free and suitable for your dietary needs.

5. Follow each recipe carefully, paying attention to measurements, cooking times, and instructions for gluten-free substitutes. Enjoy the process of exploring delicious, celiac-friendly meals with your cookbook as your guide.

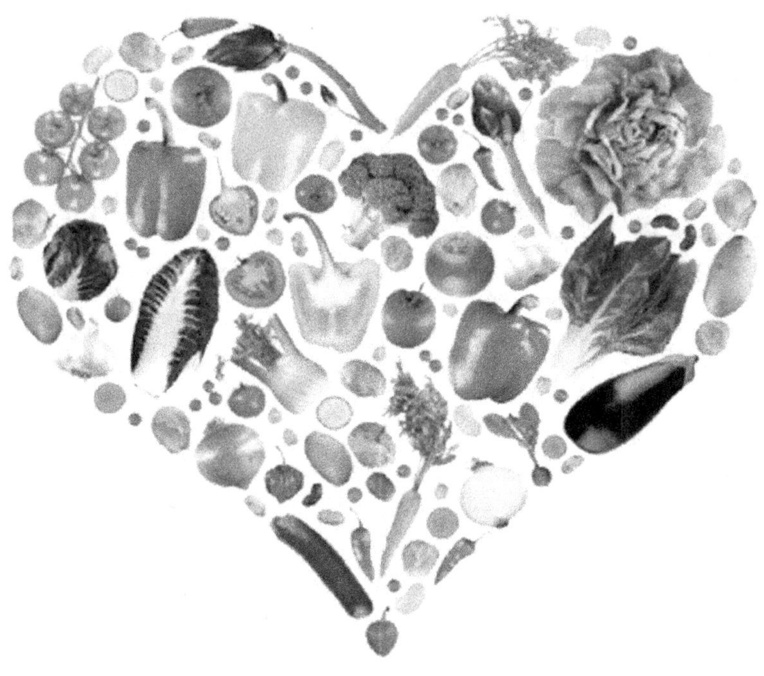

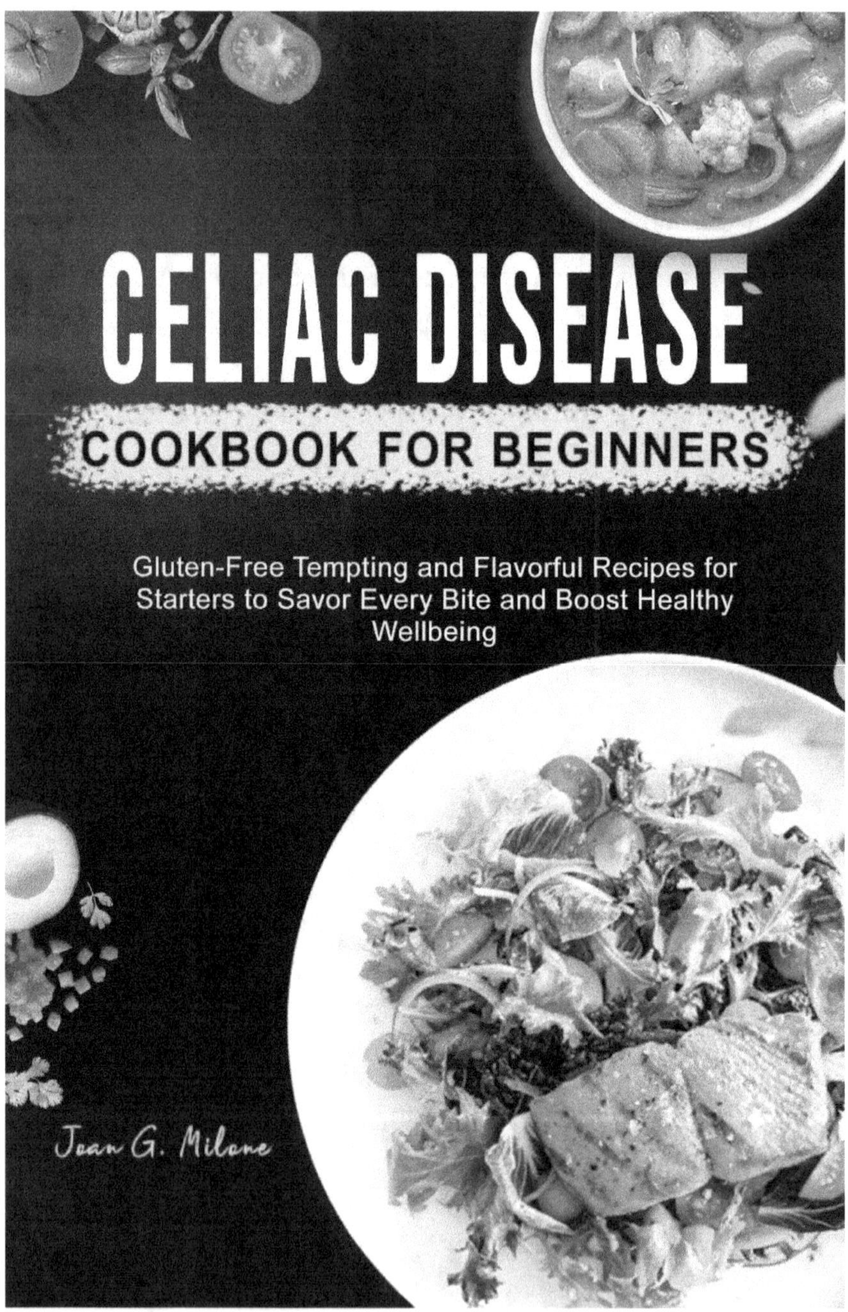

CELIAC DISEASE
COOKBOOK FOR BEGINNERS
Gluten-Free Tempting and Flavorful Recipes for Starters to Savor Every Bite and Boost Healthy Wellbeing
Jean G. Milone

Table of Contents

Introduction

Picture a time when the internet wasn't at your beck and call when finding out about celiac disease and going gluten-free meant delving into a maze of uncertainty. That's where my story begins. Back then, you couldn't just ask Siri to explain what celiac was or how to navigate a gluten-free diet. No, you had to hunt down information the old-fashioned way, through books, leaflets, and conversations.

Perhaps you learned about celiac disease after receiving your diagnosis, or perhaps someone close to you confronted this unexpected reality. Regardless matter how you got here, know that I have been in your shoes. I understand the range of emotions and problems associated with celiac disease.

Living with celiac disease is not easy. There's confusion, resentment, and even feelings of loneliness. But there's also empowerment, joy, and a ton of good cuisine to try. In this cookbook, I want to share not only tasty recipes but also the wisdom and insights I've picked up along the way.

Whether you're new to gluten-free cooking or an experienced pro, this book will be your best friend in the kitchen. It's jam-packed with comfort, inspiration, and practical advice to help you embrace gluten-free living with ease.

So, let's create some magic together! Turn the pages, test the recipes, and let's make every meal a feast of taste and nourishment. Welcome to the Celiac Disease Cookbook for Beginners, where delicious cuisine and great company go hand in hand.

Understanding Celiac Disease

Understanding celiac disease is critical for everyone living with this autoimmune disorder. Celiac illness is caused by consuming gluten, a protein present in wheat, barley, and rye. When people with celiac disease consume gluten, it causes an immune reaction that destroys the lining of the small intestine, resulting in a variety of symptoms and long-term health consequences.

Celiac disease symptoms can range from digestive disorders such as bloating, diarrhea, and constipation to exhaustion, weight loss, and skin rashes. However, some people may not experience any symptoms at all, making diagnosis difficult.

Celiac illness can only be treated with a rigorous gluten-free diet. This includes avoiding all gluten-containing foods, beverages, and non-food goods such as pharmaceuticals and cosmetics. A gluten-free diet can help alleviate symptoms and prevent additional damage to the small intestine.

Individuals with celiac disease should be aware of gluten-containing products and cross-contamination hazards, both at home and when dining out. Regular follow-ups with healthcare providers are also essential for monitoring symptoms, nutrient deficits, and overall wellness.

By understanding celiac disease and its implications, you can take control of your health and lead fulfilling lives while managing this condition effectively.

The Importance of Gluten-Free Diet

Let's talk about why being gluten-free is so crucial, especially if you have celiac disease or are gluten-sensitive. When you have celiac disease, consuming gluten (found in wheat, barley, and rye) triggers a full immune system response in your body. It destroys your small intestine, causing a variety of unpleasant symptoms and long-term health problems.

Now, the only effective strategy to manage celiac disease is to follow a strict gluten-free diet. It relieves discomfort and avoids further harm to your intestines. But it's not only celiac disease; even those who don't have it feel better when they avoid gluten. They may be gluten-sensitive or simply find that gluten causes bloating or fatigue.

So, whether you have celiac disease, gluten sensitivity, or are simply curious about the gluten-free lifestyle, understanding the significance of going gluten-free is essential. It's all about taking control of your health and well-being and making decisions that make you feel your best.

Tips for Gluten-Free Cooking and Baking

Here are some handy tips to make your gluten-free cooking and baking adventures a success:

1. **Start with the Right Ingredients**: Use gluten-free flours like rice flour, almond flour, or coconut flour for baking. Make sure your other ingredients, like spices, baking powder, and extracts, are also certified gluten-free.

2. **Experiment with Blending Flours**: Mix different gluten-free flours together to create a custom blend that works best for your recipes. This can help mimic the texture and taste of traditional baked goods.

3. **Add Binding Agents**: Since gluten provides structure in baking, you'll need to add binding agents like xanthan gum or guar gum to your recipes. These helps hold everything together and prevent crumbly results.

4. **Measure Accurately**: Use measuring cups and spoons specifically designed for dry and wet ingredients to ensure accuracy. Gluten-free flours can be finicky, so precise measurements are crucial for consistent results.

5. **Watch Your Liquid Ratios**: Gluten-free flours tend to absorb more moisture than wheat flour. Adjust your liquid ratios accordingly to prevent your baked goods from becoming too dry or too dense.

6. **Incorporate Moisture-Rich Ingredients**: Add moisture-rich ingredients like mashed bananas, applesauce, yogurt, or sour cream to your recipes to keep your baked goods moist and tender.

7. **Let it Rest**: Allow your gluten-free batters and doughs to rest for a few minutes before baking. This gives the flours time to absorb the liquids and helps improve the texture of your final product.

8. **Practice Patience**: Gluten-free baking often requires a bit of trial and error. Don't get discouraged if your first few attempts don't turn out perfectly. Keep experimenting and refining your techniques.

9. **Keep it Clean**: Avoid cross-contamination by thoroughly cleaning your kitchen surfaces, utensils, and equipment before using them for gluten-free cooking and baking.

10. **Get Creative**: Embrace the versatility of gluten-free ingredients and experiment with new recipes and flavor combinations. You might just discover some delicious new favorites along the way!

With these tips in your arsenal, you'll be well-equipped to tackle gluten-free cooking and baking with confidence and creativity.

Happy Cooking!

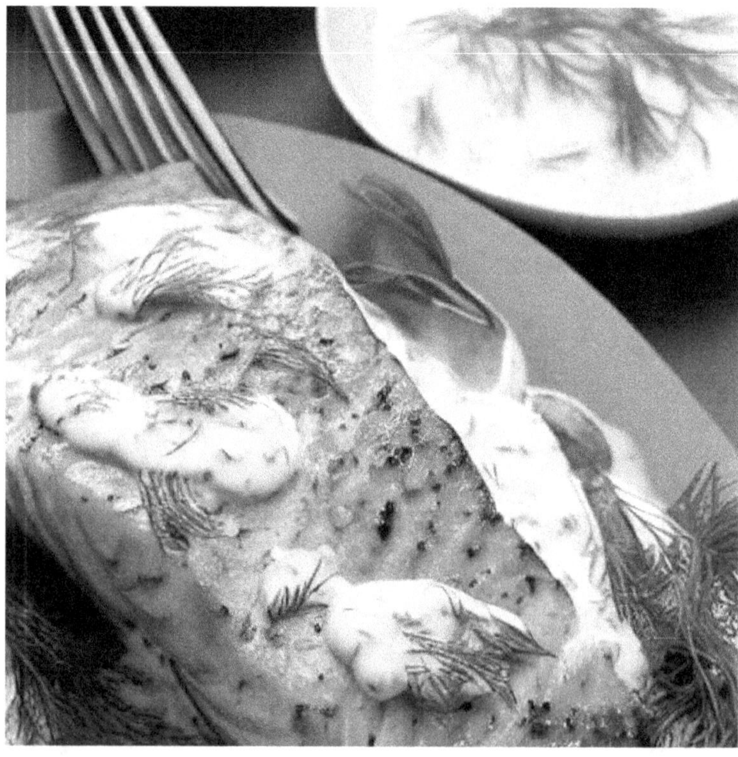

Chapter 1: Breakfasts

Start your day off properly with delicious and fulfilling gluten-free breakfast alternatives that will energize your morning and get your day started. From hearty and nutritious meals to quick and convenient grab-and-go options, we have something for everyone. Whether you want traditional favorites like pancakes and waffles or want to try something different like savory breakfast bowls or revitalizing smoothie bowls, our Breakfasts chapter has you covered. Prepare to rise and shine with delectable recipes that demonstrate how gluten-free breakfasts can be both healthful and delicious.

Quinoa and Chia Porridge

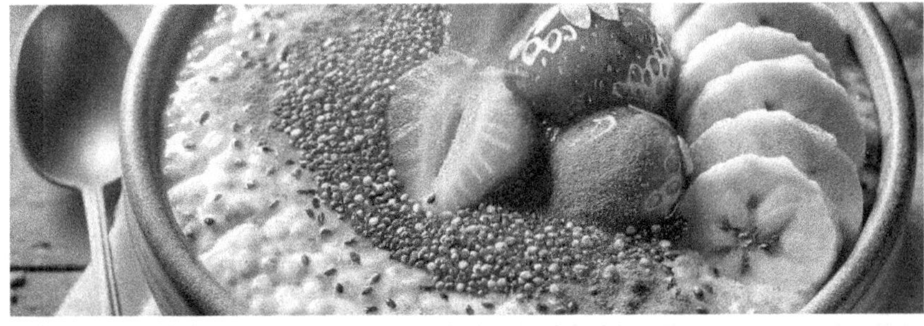

Ingredients:

- 1 cup quinoa, rinsed
- 2 cups almond milk (or any milk of choice)
- 2 tablespoons chia seeds
- 1 tablespoon maple syrup (adjust to taste)
- 1 teaspoon vanilla extract
- Pinch of salt
- Fresh fruits, nuts, and seeds for topping

Preparation:

1. Combine quinoa, almond milk, chia seeds, maple syrup, vanilla extract, and a pinch of salt in a medium saucepan.

2. Bring the mixture to a boil, then reduce heat and simmer, covered, for about 15 minutes, or until the quinoa is cooked and the mixture has thickened.

3. Stir occasionally to prevent sticking. Add more milk if needed for desired consistency.

4. Serve warm, topped with your choice of fresh fruits, nuts, and seeds.

Cooking Time: Approximately 20 minutes.

Nutritional Values (per serving, without toppings):

- Calories: ~250
- Protein: ~8 grams
- Fat: ~5 grams (varies with toppings)

- Carbohydrates: ~40 grams
- Fiber: ~6 grams

Rating: ★★★★★

This porridge is highly rated for its balance of proteins, healthy fats, and fibers, making it an excellent gluten-free choice to fuel your day.

Gluten-Free Oatmeal Pancakes

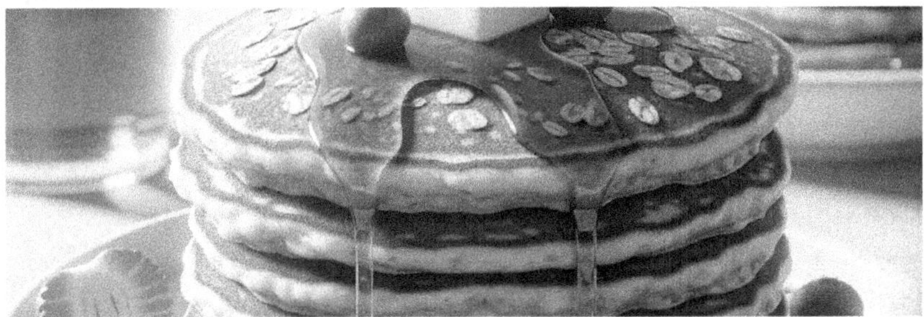

Ingredients:

- 1 cup gluten-free oats
- 1 banana
- 2 eggs
- 1/2 cup almond milk (or any milk of choice)
- 1 teaspoon baking powder
- 1/2 teaspoon vanilla extract
- Pinch of salt
- Cooking spray or butter for the pan

Preparation:

1. Blend the oats in a blender until they reach a flour-like consistency.

2. Add the banana, eggs, almond milk, baking powder, vanilla extract, and salt to the blender. Blend until smooth.

3. Heat a non-stick pan over medium heat and lightly grease with cooking spray or butter.

4. Pour batter onto the pan to form pancakes of your desired size. Cook until bubbles form on the surface, then flip and cook until golden brown.

5. Serve hot with your favorite toppings.

Cooking Time: Approximately 15 minutes.

Nutritional Values (per serving, without toppings):

- Calories: ~280
- Protein: ~11 grams
- Fat: ~7 grams
- Carbohydrates: ~44 grams
- Fiber: ~6 grams

Rating: ★★★★★

These pancakes are beloved for their heartiness and versatility. They're packed with fiber and protein, making them a fantastic gluten-free option to kickstart your day.

Almond Flour Waffles

Ingredients:

- 2 cups almond flour
- 3 eggs
- 1/2 cup water (or almond milk for richer flavor)

- 1/4 cup vegetable oil or melted butter
- 2 tablespoons erythritol (or sweetener of choice)
- 1 teaspoon baking powder
- 1/2 teaspoon vanilla extract
- Pinch of salt

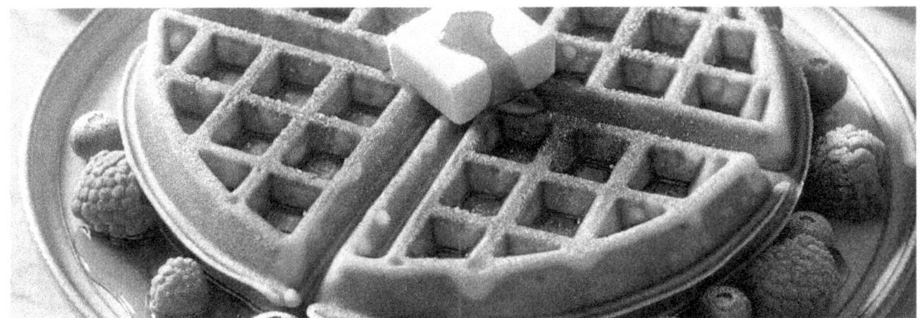

Preparation:

1. In a large bowl, whisk together the almond flour, baking powder, erythritol, and salt.

2. In another bowl, beat the eggs, then mix in the water (or almond milk), vegetable oil, and vanilla extract.

3. Combine wet and dry ingredients, mixing until smooth.

4. Preheat your waffle iron and lightly grease it with oil or butter.

5. Pour enough batter into the iron to just cover the waffle grid.

6. Close the lid and cook until the waffle is golden and crisp, about 3-5 minutes.

7. Serve warm with your favorite toppings.

Cooking Time: Approximately 5 minutes per waffle.

Nutritional Values (per waffle, without toppings):

- Calories: ~300
- Protein: ~10 grams
- Fat: ~25 grams
- Carbohydrates: ~12 grams
- Fiber: ~3 grams

Rating: ★★★★★

Almond Flour Waffles are celebrated for their delicious taste and satisfying texture, offering a fantastic start to the day for those following a gluten-free or low-carb diet.

Breakfast Quiche with Gluten-Free Crust

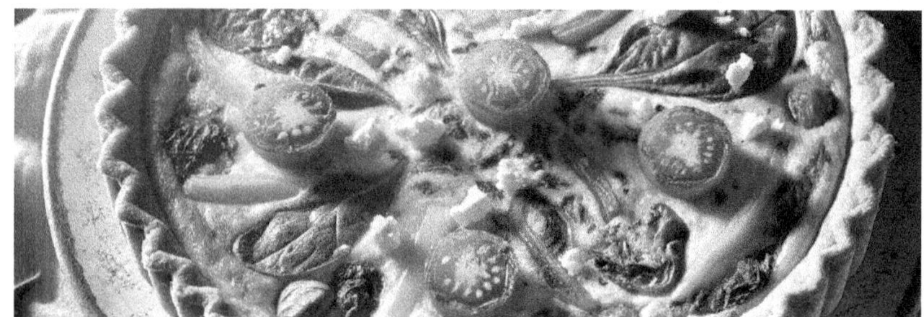

Ingredients:

- For the crust:
    - 1.5 cups almond flour
    - 1/4 cup coconut oil (solid)
    - 1 egg
    - Pinch of salt
- For the filling:
    - 6 eggs
    - 1/2 cup milk (dairy or non-dairy)
    - 1 cup cooked spinach

- 1/2 cup diced ham (optional, ensure gluten-free)
- 1/2 cup shredded cheese (your choice)
- Salt and pepper to taste

Preparation:

1. Preheat oven to 350°F (175°C).

2. Mix almond flour and salt for the crust. Add coconut oil and 1 egg, mixing until dough forms. Press into a 9-inch pie pan.

3. Bake crust for 10 minutes. Remove from oven.

4. Whisk together eggs and milk. Stir in spinach, ham, and half the cheese. Season with salt and pepper.

5. Pour the filling into the pre-baked crust. Top with the remaining cheese.

6. Bake for 35-40 minutes, or until the quiche is set and the top is golden.

7. Let cool for a few minutes before serving.

Cooking Time: 50 minutes total (10 minutes for crust, 40 minutes for quiche).

Nutritional Values (per slice, based on 8 slices, without optional ham):

- Calories: ~280
- Protein: ~14 grams
- Fat: ~23 grams
- Carbohydrates: ~8 grams
- Fiber: ~3 grams

Rating: ★★★★★

This Breakfast Quiche with Gluten-Free Crust is highly rated for its versatility, ease of preparation, and delicious taste. It's a great option for a nutritious, satisfying meal that's both gluten-free and customizable to your dietary needs or preferences.

Avocado Toast on Gluten-Free Bread

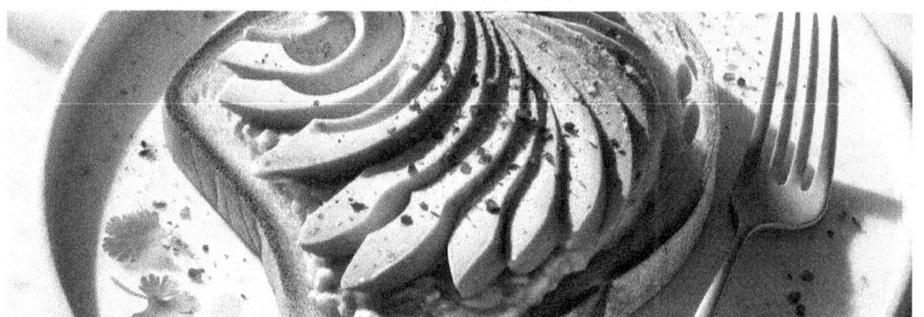

Ingredients:

- 2 slices of gluten-free bread
- 1 ripe avocado
- Salt and pepper to taste
- Optional toppings: sliced tomatoes, radishes, sprouts, poached egg, red pepper flakes

Preparation:

1. Toast the gluten-free bread slices to your liking.

2. Mash the avocado in a bowl with a fork. Season with salt and pepper.

3. Spread the mashed avocado evenly over the toasted bread slices.

4. Add any optional toppings you prefer.

Cooking Time: About 5 minutes, depending on your toaster.

Nutritional Values (per serving, without optional toppings):

- Calories: ~300
- Protein: ~5 grams
- Fat: ~20 grams (mostly healthy fats from the avocado)
- Carbohydrates: ~30 grams
- Fiber: ~7 grams

Rating: ★★★★★

Avocado Toast on Gluten-Free Bread is celebrated for its ease of preparation, health benefits, and delicious taste. It's a flexible dish that can be tailored with various toppings to suit your mood or dietary requirements.

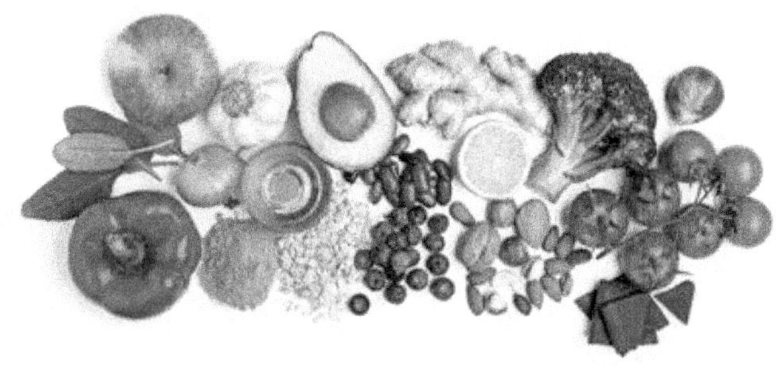

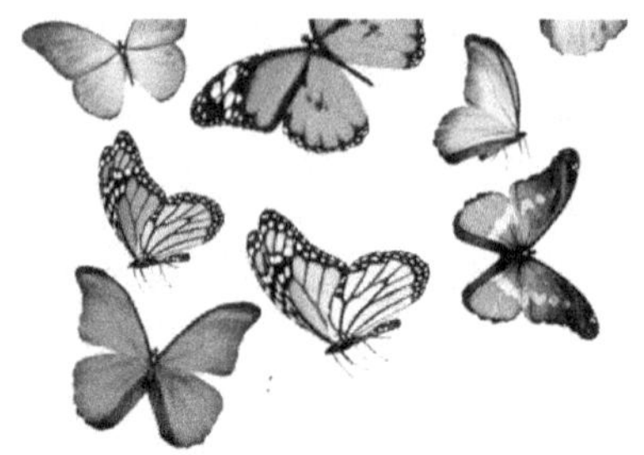

Embrace vibrant veggies, fruits, and whole grains as your allies. Your journey to reverse celiac disease starts with nourishing choices. Let wholesome foods be your path to healing and vitality.

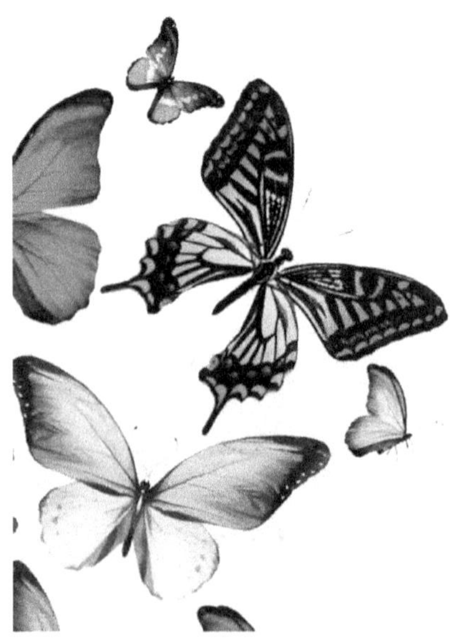

Chapter 2: Lunch

Say goodbye to monotonous midday meals and hello to a world of delectable and filling gluten-free lunch alternatives. Whether you're looking for simple packed lunches for work or school, robust salads for a refreshing dinner, or warm soups and sandwiches for a comfortable lunch at home, we've got you covered. Get ready to up your lunch game with this collection of delicious gluten-free meals that will keep you satiated and fueled for the rest of the day.

Gluten-Free Pasta Salad

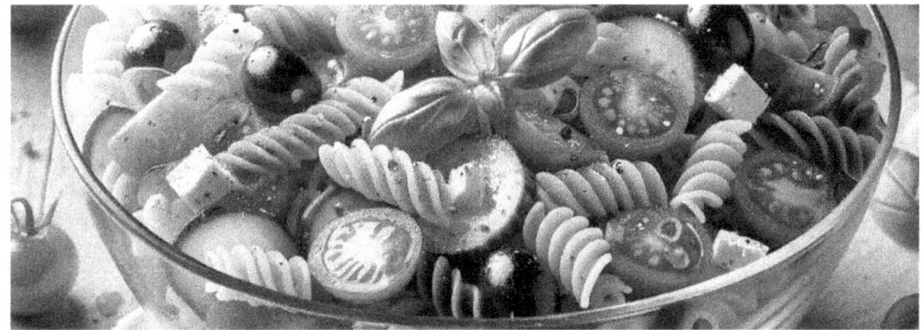

Ingredients:

- 8 ounces gluten-free pasta (e.g., penne, fusilli)
- 1 cup cherry tomatoes, halved
- 1/2 cup cucumber, diced
- 1/2 cup black olives, sliced
- 1/4 cup red onion, thinly sliced
- 1/2 cup feta cheese, crumbled
- 1/4 cup olive oil
- 2 tablespoons red wine vinegar
- 1 teaspoon dried oregano
- Salt and pepper to taste

Preparation:

1. Cook the gluten-free pasta according to package instructions, then rinse under cold water and drain.

2. In a large bowl, combine the cooked pasta, cherry tomatoes, cucumber, black olives, red onion, and feta cheese.

3. In a small bowl, whisk together the olive oil, red wine vinegar, oregano, salt, and pepper to create the dressing.

4. Pour the dressing over the pasta mixture and toss until everything is evenly coated.

5. Chill in the refrigerator for at least 1 hour before serving to enhance flavors.

Cooking Time: 15 minutes for pasta cooking; 1 hour for chilling.

Nutritional Values (per serving, based on 6 servings):

- Calories: ~250
- Protein: ~5 grams
- Fat: ~14 grams
- Carbohydrates: ~28 grams
- Fiber: ~2 grams

Rating: ★★★★★

This Gluten-Free Pasta Salad scores high for its delicious taste, ease of preparation, and adaptability to various dietary preferences. It's a colorful, nutritious dish that's perfect for any occasion.

Quinoa Tabbouleh

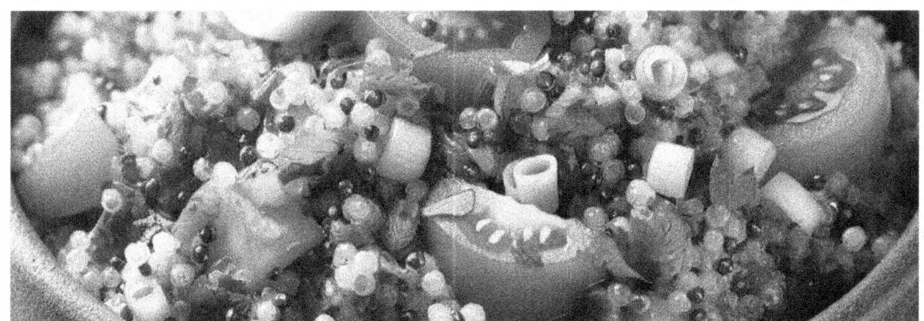

Ingredients:

- 1 cup quinoa
- 2 cups water
- 1 cup fresh parsley, finely chopped
- 1/2 cup fresh mint, finely chopped
- 1/2 cup cucumber, diced
- 1 cup tomatoes, diced
- 1/4 cup lemon juice
- 1/4 cup olive oil
- Salt and pepper to taste

Preparation:

1. Rinse quinoa under cold water. In a pot, bring 2 cups of water to a boil. Add quinoa, reduce heat, cover, and simmer for about 15 minutes or until water is absorbed. Let it cool.

2. In a large bowl, combine cooled quinoa, parsley, mint, cucumber, and tomatoes.

3. In a small bowl, whisk together lemon juice, olive oil, salt, and pepper to make the dressing.

4. Pour the dressing over the quinoa mixture and toss to combine thoroughly.

5. Refrigerate for at least 30 minutes before serving to let the flavors meld.

Cooking Time: 15 minutes for cooking quinoa; 30 minutes for chilling.

Nutritional Values (per serving, based on 6 servings):

- Calories: ~200
- Protein: ~4 grams
- Fat: ~10 grams
- Carbohydrates: ~23 grams
- Fiber: ~3 grams

Rating: ★★★★★

Quinoa Tabbouleh is celebrated for its fresh flavors, health benefits, and versatility. It's a perfect dish for anyone looking for a nutritious, gluten-free option that doesn't compromise on taste.

Grilled Chicken Wrap (Gluten-Free Tortilla)

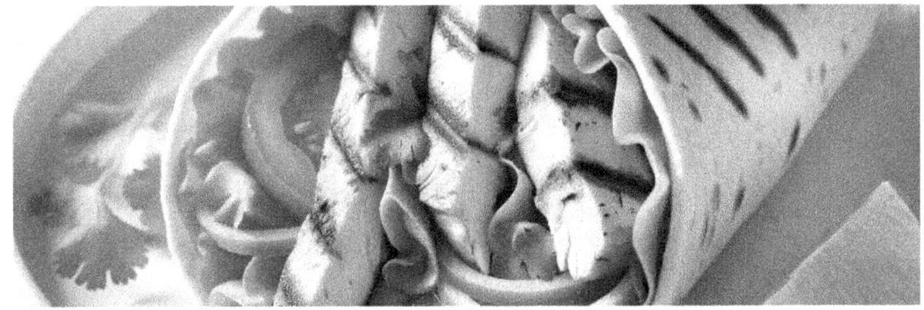

Ingredients:

- 2 gluten-free tortillas
- 2 chicken breasts, grilled and sliced
- 1/2 avocado, sliced
- 1/4 cup shredded lettuce
- 1/4 cup diced tomatoes
- 2 tablespoons ranch dressing (ensure gluten-free)
- Salt and pepper to taste

Preparation:

1. Grill chicken breasts seasoned with salt and pepper until fully cooked and juicy, about 6-8 minutes per side depending on thickness.

2. Warm the gluten-free tortillas in a dry pan for about 30 seconds on each side to make them pliable.

3. Lay out the tortillas and evenly distribute the grilled chicken, avocado slices, shredded lettuce, and diced tomatoes onto each tortilla.

4. Drizzle with ranch dressing and season with salt and pepper to taste.

5. Carefully roll up the tortillas, folding in the sides to enclose the filling.

6. Cut in half and serve immediately.

Cooking Time: About 20 minutes.

Nutritional Values (per wrap):

- Calories: ~400
- Protein: ~35 grams
- Fat: ~20 grams
- Carbohydrates: ~25 grams
- Fiber: ~5 grams

Rating: ★★★★★

This Grilled Chicken Wrap in a Gluten-Free Tortilla is highly rated for its delicious taste, balance of nutrients, and simplicity in preparation. It's a fantastic, quick meal that satisfies without feeling heavy.

Stuffed Bell Peppers

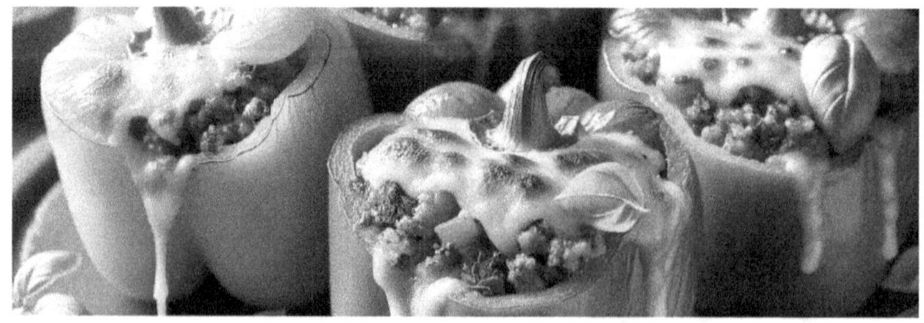

Ingredients:

- 4 large bell peppers, any color
- 1 pound ground turkey (or beef, for a non-vegetarian option)
- 1 cup cooked quinoa or rice (ensure gluten-free if using packaged)
- 1 cup tomato sauce
- 1/2 cup onion, diced
- 1 garlic clove, minced
- 1 teaspoon cumin
- 1 teaspoon paprika
- Salt and pepper to taste
- 1/2 cup shredded cheese (optional, for topping)

Preparation:

1. Preheat oven to 375°F (190°C).
2. Cut the tops off the bell peppers and remove seeds. Place in a baking dish.
3. In a skillet, cook the ground turkey with onion and garlic until browned. Season with cumin, paprika, salt, and pepper.
4. Stir in the cooked quinoa or rice and tomato sauce until well combined.
5. Stuff the mixture into the bell peppers, top with shredded cheese if using.
6. Cover with foil and bake for 30 minutes. Uncover and bake for an additional 10 minutes, or until the peppers are tender and the cheese is bubbly.
7. Serve hot.

Cooking Time: 40 minutes.

Nutritional Values (per stuffed pepper, using turkey and quinoa, without cheese):

- Calories: ~250
- Protein: ~21 grams
- Fat: ~7 grams
- Carbohydrates: ~27 grams
- Fiber: ~5 grams

Rating: ★★★★★

Stuffed Bell Peppers are a versatile dish that can be customized with various fillings and spices. They're well-loved for their vibrant presentation, rich flavors, and balanced nutrition profile.

Butternut Squash Soup

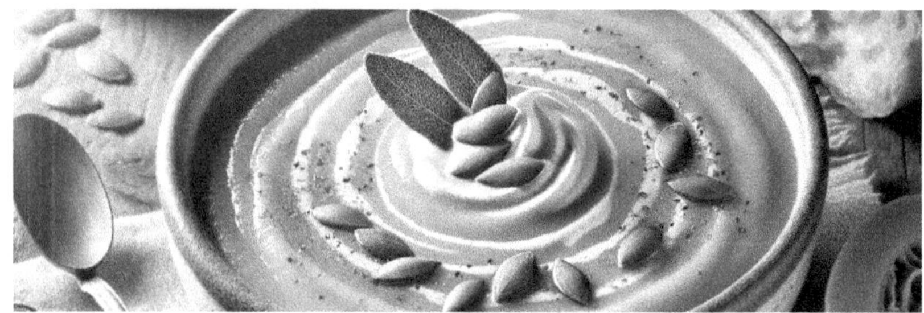

Ingredients:

- 1 large butternut squash, peeled, seeded, and cubed
- 1 onion, chopped
- 2 garlic cloves, minced
- 4 cups vegetable broth
- 1 teaspoon thyme
- Salt and pepper to taste
- 1 cup coconut milk (for creaminess)
- Olive oil for sautéing

Preparation:

1. In a large pot, heat olive oil over medium heat. Add onion and garlic, sauté until soft.

2. Add butternut squash, vegetable broth, thyme, salt, and pepper. Bring to a boil, then simmer until squash is tender, about 20 minutes.

3. Use an immersion blender to puree the soup until smooth. Stir in coconut milk and adjust seasoning as needed.

4. Simmer for an additional 5 minutes. Serve warm.

Cooking Time: About 30 minutes.

Nutritional Values (per serving, based on 4 servings):

- Calories: ~180
- Protein: ~2 grams
- Fat: ~9 grams (mostly from coconut milk)
- Carbohydrates: ~25 grams
- Fiber: ~5 grams

Rating: ★★★★★

Butternut Squash Soup is praised for its smooth texture, rich flavors, and nutritional benefits. It's a delicious way to enjoy a serving of vegetables, making it a hit for both taste and health.

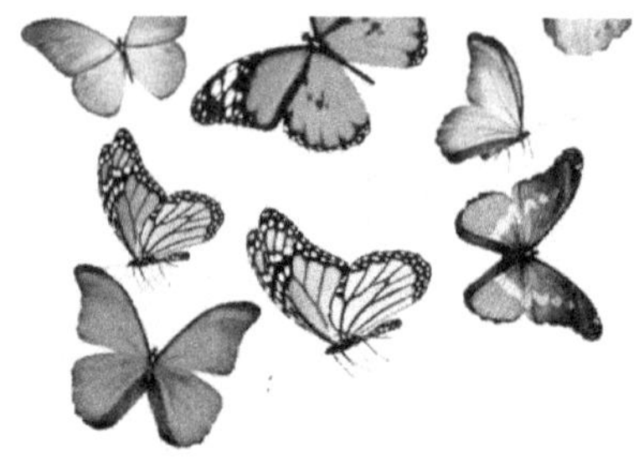

Fill your plate with nature's bounty – colorful fruits, leafy greens, and nutrient-rich grains. Every bite fuels your body's fight against celiac disease. Trust in the power of wholesome nutrition.

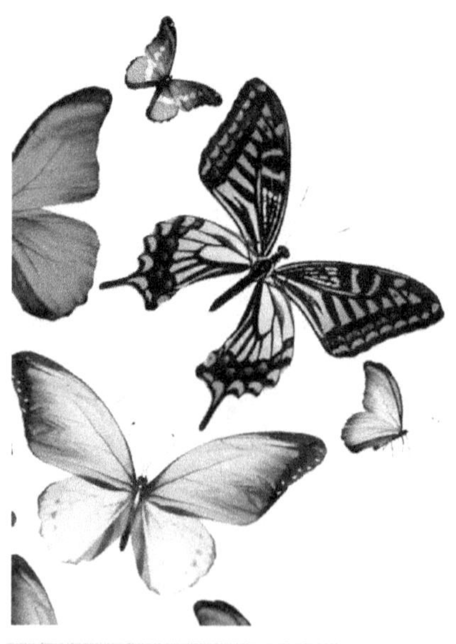

Chapter 3: Dinner

Prepare to transform your evening meals into unique dining experiences with our collection of delicious gluten-free supper recipes. Our Dinner chapter has something for everyone, whether you're entertaining a large crowd or spending a relaxing evening at home. Discover new flavors, try new cuisines, and enjoy healthful, handmade meals that are both delicious and gluten-free. With simple directions and plenty of tips and tricks, you'll be preparing restaurant-quality meals in no time. So, grab your apron and prepare to dazzle your family and friends with our delectable gluten-free supper recipes.

Gluten-Free Pizza with a Cauliflower Crust

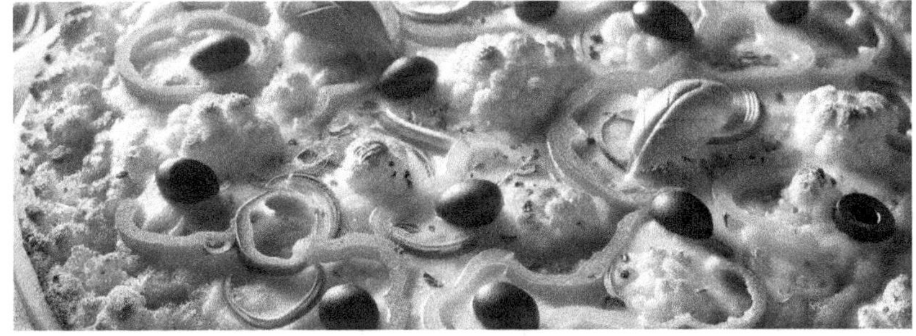

Ingredients:

- 1 medium head of cauliflower, riced
- 1 egg, beaten
- 1/2 cup shredded mozzarella cheese
- 1 teaspoon oregano
- Salt and pepper to taste
- 1/2 cup tomato sauce
- 1 cup toppings of choice (e.g., vegetables, cooked chicken, more cheese)

Preparation:

1. Preheat your oven to 400°F (200°C). Line a baking sheet with parchment paper.

2. Microwave the riced cauliflower for about 5 minutes, let it cool, then squeeze out as much moisture as possible using a kitchen towel.

3. Mix the cauliflower with the egg, mozzarella, oregano, salt, and pepper.

4. Press the mixture onto the baking sheet, forming a thin, round pizza base.

5. Bake for 20 minutes or until golden.

6. Spread tomato sauce over the baked crust, add your toppings, and sprinkle with additional cheese.

7. Bake for another 10 minutes, or until the toppings are hot and the cheese is melted.

Cooking Time: Approximately 30 minutes.

Nutritional Values (per serving, based on 4 servings without specific toppings):

- Calories: ~150
- Protein: ~10 grams
- Fat: ~7 grams
- Carbohydrates: ~10 grams
- Fiber: ~3 grams

Rating: ★★★★★

This Gluten-Free Pizza with a Cauliflower Crust is celebrated for its innovative use of cauliflower, providing a healthier, tasty base that's perfect for those looking to reduce gluten and carbs in their diet.

Baked Salmon with Dill Sauce

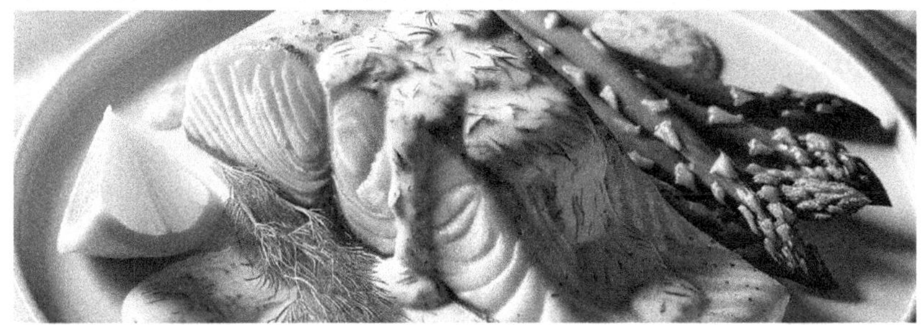

Ingredients:

- 4 salmon fillets
- 2 tablespoons olive oil
- Salt and pepper to taste

- 1 lemon, sliced (for garnish)
- **For the Dill Sauce:**
  - 1/2 cup Greek yogurt
  - 2 tablespoons fresh dill, chopped
- 1 tablespoon lemon juice
- 1 garlic clove, minced
- Salt and pepper to taste

Preparation:

1. Preheat your oven to 375°F (190°C). Line a baking sheet with foil or parchment paper.

2. Place salmon fillets on the baking sheet. Drizzle with olive oil, season with salt and pepper.

3. Bake for 12-15 minutes, or until the salmon is cooked through and flakes easily with a fork.

4. While the salmon bakes, mix together Greek yogurt, dill, lemon juice, garlic, salt, and pepper in a bowl to make the sauce.

5. Serve the baked salmon with the dill sauce and garnish with lemon slices.

Cooking Time: 15 minutes.

Nutritional Values (per serving):

- Calories: ~300
- Protein: ~23 grams

- Fat: ~20 grams (mostly healthy fats from salmon and olive oil)
- Carbohydrates: ~3 grams
- Fiber: ~0 grams

Rating: ★★★★★

Baked Salmon with Dill Sauce scores high for its ease of preparation, delicious taste, and nutritional benefits, making it a favorite for a quick, healthy meal.

Vegetable Stir-Fry with Gluten-Free Soy Sauce

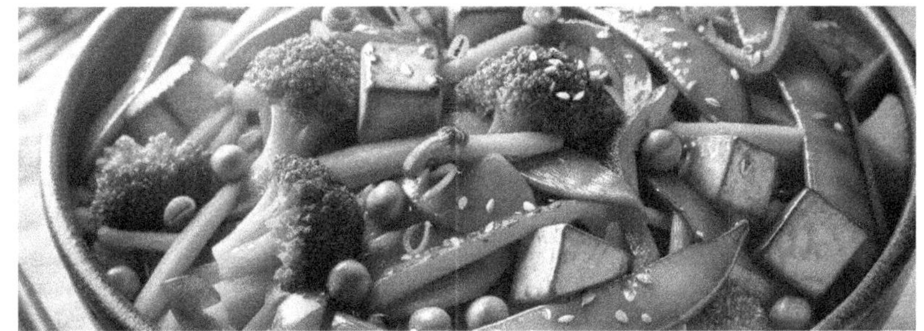

Ingredients:

- 2 tablespoons olive oil
- 2 cups mixed vegetables (e.g., bell peppers, broccoli, snap peas, carrots)
- 1 onion, sliced
- 2 garlic cloves, minced
- 1/4 cup gluten-free soy sauce
- 1 tablespoon sesame oil
- 1 teaspoon ginger, grated
- Salt and pepper to taste
- Optional: tofu, chicken, or beef for added protein

Preparation:

1. Heat olive oil in a large pan or wok over medium-high heat.

2. Add onion and garlic, sauté for 2 minutes until fragrant.

3. Add the mixed vegetables and cook for 5-7 minutes, stirring frequently, until they are just tender but still crisp.

4. If adding protein, ensure it's cooked through at this stage.

5. Lower the heat, and stir in the gluten-free soy sauce, sesame oil, and ginger. Cook for another 2 minutes, allowing the flavors to blend.

6. Season with salt and pepper to taste. Serve hot.

Cooking Time: About 15 minutes.

Nutritional Values (per serving, vegetables only):

- Calories: ~150
- Protein: ~3 grams
- Fat: ~10 grams
- Carbohydrates: ~12 grams
- Fiber: ~3 grams

Rating: ★★★★★

This Vegetable Stir-Fry with Gluten-Free Soy Sauce is highly rated for its simplicity, flavor, and adaptability to include various vegetables or proteins. It's a go-to for a healthy, satisfying meal that's quick to prepare.

Grilled Steak with Chimichurri Sauce

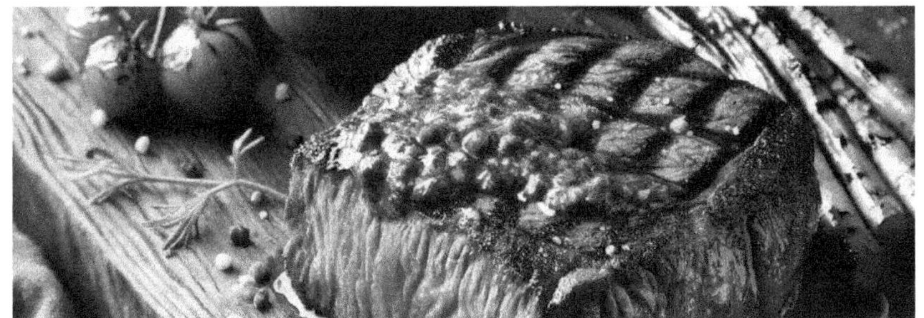

Ingredients:

- 2 lbs flank steak
- Salt and pepper to taste
- **For the Chimichurri Sauce:**
    - 1 cup fresh parsley, finely chopped
    - 1/4 cup fresh cilantro, finely chopped
- 3 cloves garlic, minced
- 1/2 cup olive oil
- 2 tablespoons red wine vinegar
- 1 teaspoon red pepper flakes
- Salt and pepper to taste

Preparation:

1. Season the flank steak with salt and pepper.

2. Preheat your grill to medium-high heat. Grill the steak for 5-7 minutes per side for medium-rare, or until it reaches your desired doneness.

3. For the chimichurri sauce, combine parsley, cilantro, garlic, olive oil, red wine vinegar, red pepper flakes, salt, and pepper in a bowl. Stir well.

4. Slice the steak across the grain and serve with the chimichurri sauce drizzled on top.

Cooking Time: 30 minutes.

Nutritional Values (per serving):

- Calories: ~350
- Protein: ~25 grams
- Fat: ~25 grams
- Carbohydrates: ~2 grams
- Fiber: ~1 gram
- Sodium: ~200 mg

Rating: ★★★★☆

This Grilled Steak with Chimichurri Sauce is celebrated for its robust flavors and healthful approach, catering well to those with celiac disease or anyone looking for a delicious gluten-free option.

Eggplant Parmesan with Gluten-Free Breadcrumbs

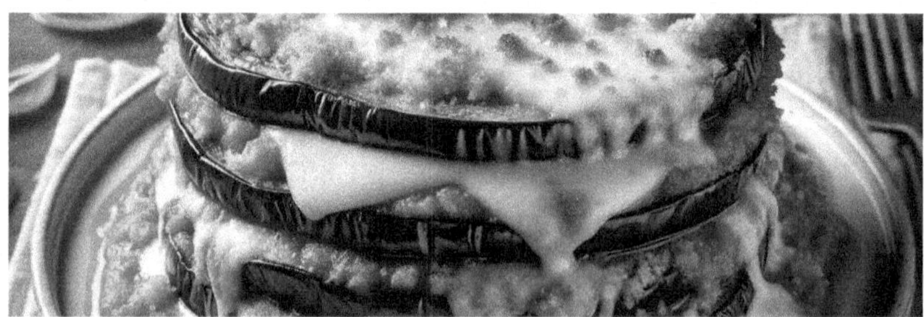

Ingredients:

- 2 large eggplants, sliced into 1/2-inch rounds
- Salt, for drawing water out of eggplant
- 2 cups gluten-free breadcrumbs
- 2 eggs, beaten
- 1/2 cup grated Parmesan cheese
- 2 cups marinara sauce, gluten-free
- 2 cups shredded mozzarella cheese
- 1 tablespoon olive oil
- Fresh basil for garnish

Preparation:

1. Sprinkle salt on the eggplant slices and let them sit for about 20 minutes to draw out moisture. Pat dry with paper towels.
2. Preheat the oven to 375°F (190°C). Grease a baking sheet with olive oil.
3. Mix gluten-free breadcrumbs with grated Parmesan cheese.
4. Dip eggplant slices in beaten eggs, then coat with breadcrumb mixture. Place on the prepared baking sheet.
5. Bake in preheated oven for 25 minutes, flipping once until golden brown.
6. In a baking dish, spread a layer of marinara sauce, place a layer of baked eggplant slices, and top with mozzarella cheese. Repeat layers.
7. Bake for an additional 20 minutes, or until cheese is bubbly and golden.

8. Garnish with fresh basil before serving.

Cooking Time: About 1 hour.

Nutritional Values (per serving):

- Calories: ~330
- Protein: ~18 grams
- Fat: ~18 grams
-
- Carbohydrates: ~24 grams
- Fiber: ~6 grams
- Sodium: ~600 mg

Rating: ★★★★★

This Eggplant Parmesan with Gluten-Free Breadcrumbs recipe offers a delightful twist on a classic, making it a perfect dish for those following a gluten-free diet without compromising on taste or texture.

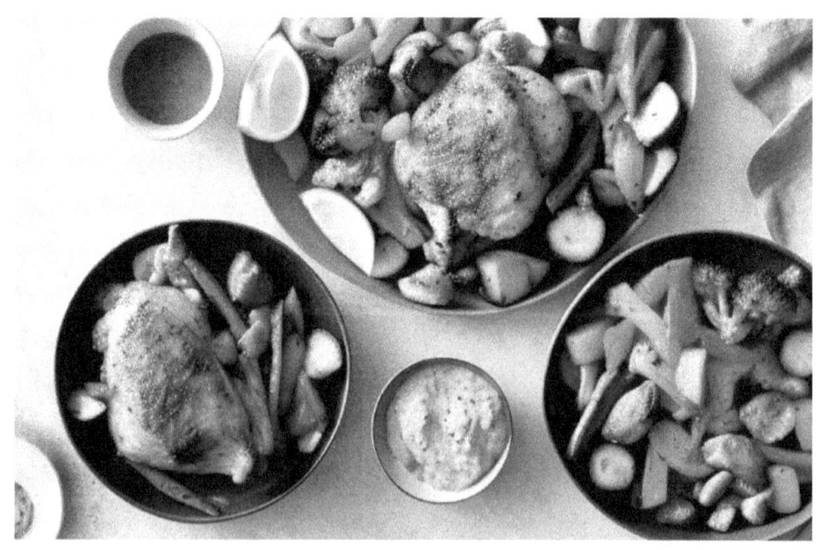

Chapter 4: Soups

Warm up your kitchen and your soul with our selection of delicious and savory gluten-free soup recipes. From creamy bisques to chunky stews, our soup recipes are packed with wholesome ingredients and bold flavors that are sure to leave you feeling nourished and satisfied. Whether you're serving up a cozy dinner for the family or looking for a quick and easy meal to enjoy on a chilly evening, our Soups chapter has you covered. So, grab a spoon and get ready to savor the goodness of homemade gluten-free soups that are guaranteed to warm you from the inside out.

Creamy Tomato Soup

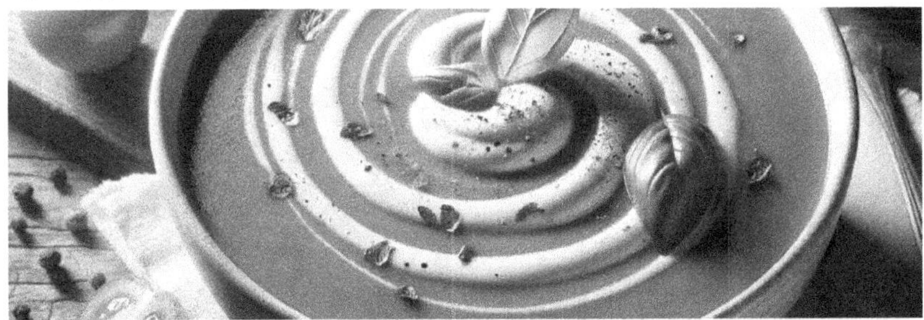

Ingredients:

- 2 tablespoons olive oil
- 1 onion, diced
- 2 garlic cloves, minced
- 1 can (28 ounces) whole peeled tomatoes, with juice
- 1 cup vegetable broth, gluten-free
- 1/2 cup heavy cream
- 2 teaspoons sugar (optional, to taste)
- Salt and pepper to taste
- Fresh basil leaves, for garnish

Preparation:

1. Heat olive oil in a large pot over medium heat. Add onion and garlic, and sauté until soft, about 5 minutes.

2. Add whole peeled tomatoes (with juice) and vegetable broth. Bring to a simmer.

3. Use an immersion blender to blend the soup until smooth (or transfer to a blender, then return to pot).

4. Stir in heavy cream and sugar (if using). Season with salt and pepper.

5. Simmer for an additional 10 minutes. Adjust seasoning if necessary.

6. Serve hot, garnished with fresh basil leaves.

Cooking Time: About 30 minutes.

Nutritional Values (per serving):

- Calories: ~200
- Protein: ~3 grams
- Fat: ~15 grams
- Carbohydrates: ~15 grams
- Fiber: ~3 grams
- Sodium: ~700 mg

Rating: ★★★★☆

This Creamy Tomato Soup, with its rich flavor and velvety texture, is both comforting and satisfying. It's a simple yet delicious option for anyone, especially those adhering to a gluten-free diet.

Carrot and Ginger Soup

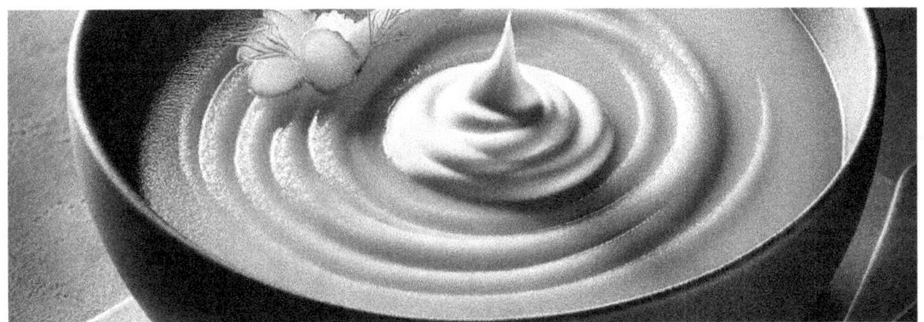

Ingredients:

- 1 tablespoon olive oil
- 1 onion, chopped
- 2 cloves garlic, minced
- 2 tablespoons fresh ginger, grated
- 1 pound carrots, peeled and chopped
- 4 cups vegetable broth, gluten-free
- Salt and pepper to taste
- Coconut milk for garnish (optional)

Preparation:

1. In a large pot, heat olive oil over medium heat. Add onion and garlic, cooking until softened, about 5 minutes.

2. Stir in ginger and carrots, and cook for another 2 minutes.

3. Pour in the vegetable broth and bring to a boil. Reduce heat and simmer until carrots are tender, about 20 minutes.

4. Use an immersion blender to purée the soup until smooth. Season with salt and pepper.

5. Serve hot, drizzled with coconut milk if desired.

Cooking Time: About 45 minutes.

Nutritional Values (per serving):

- Calories: ~120
- Protein: ~2 grams
- Fat: ~5 grams
- Carbohydrates: ~17 grams
- Fiber: ~4 grams
- Sodium: ~500 mg

Rating: ★★★★☆

This Carrot and Ginger Soup combines the sweetness of carrots with the warmth of ginger, resulting in a comforting and healthful dish perfect for any season. Its vibrant color and creamy texture make it a delightful gluten-free option.

Chicken and Rice Soup

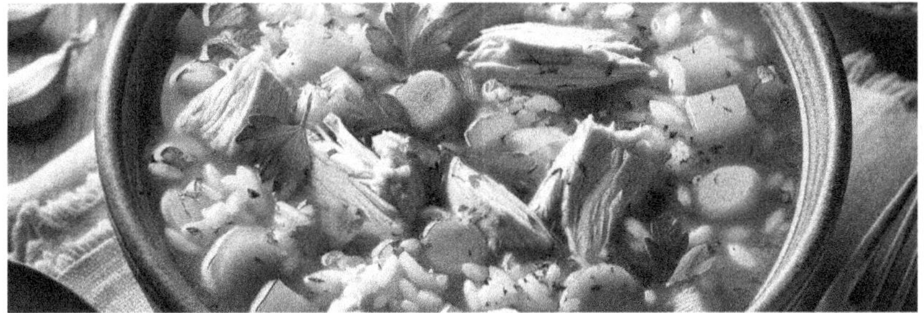

Ingredients:

- 1 tablespoon olive oil
- 1 onion, diced
- 2 carrots, peeled and diced
- 2 celery stalks, diced
- 2 garlic cloves, minced
- 1 pound chicken breast, cubed
- 6 cups chicken broth, gluten-free
- 1 cup white rice, rinsed
- Salt and pepper to taste
- Fresh parsley, chopped for garnish

Preparation:

1. Heat olive oil in a large pot over medium heat. Add onion, carrots, celery, and garlic. Sauté until vegetables are softened, about 5 minutes.

2. Add the cubed chicken to the pot and cook until no longer pink, about 5-7 minutes.

3. Pour in the chicken broth and bring to a simmer. Add the rinsed rice, and season with salt and pepper.

4. Cover and simmer on low heat until the rice is cooked and the chicken is tender, about 20 minutes.

5. Adjust seasoning to taste. Serve hot, garnished with fresh parsley.

Cooking Time: 40 minutes.

Nutritional Values (per serving):

- Calories: ~250
- Protein: ~20 grams
- Fat: ~5 grams
- Carbohydrates: ~30 grams
- Fiber: ~2 grams
- Sodium: ~700 mg

Rating: ★★★★☆

This Chicken and Rice Soup is a wholesome and comforting meal, perfect for a cold day or when you're in need of some home-cooked nourishment.

Broccoli Cheddar Soup

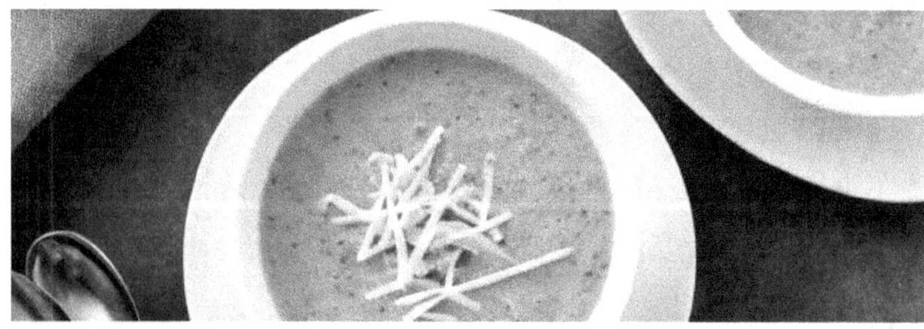

Ingredients:

- 1 tablespoon olive oil
- 1 onion, chopped

- 2 garlic cloves, minced
- 4 cups broccoli florets
- 3 cups vegetable broth, gluten-free

- 1 cup heavy cream
- 2 cups shredded cheddar cheese
- Salt and pepper to taste

Preparation:

1. In a large pot, heat olive oil over medium heat. Add onion and garlic, sautéing until softened, about 5 minutes.

2. Add broccoli and vegetable broth. Bring to a boil, then reduce heat and simmer until broccoli is tender, about 10 minutes.

3. Use an immersion blender to slightly puree the soup, leaving some broccoli chunks for texture.

4. Stir in the heavy cream and shredded cheddar cheese until the cheese is melted and the soup is heated through. Season with salt and pepper.

5. Serve hot, adjusting seasoning as needed.

Cooking Time: 30 minutes.

Nutritional Values (per serving):

- Calories: ~400
- Protein: ~15 grams
- Fat: ~34 grams

- Carbohydrates: ~10 grams
- Fiber: ~2 grams
- Sodium: ~800 mg

Rating: ★★★★☆

This Broccoli Cheddar Soup is rich, creamy, and packed with flavor. A comforting classic that's easy to prepare, it's perfect for those chilly days or when you're craving something hearty and satisfying. This gluten-free version ensures everyone can enjoy this delicious dish without compromise.

Lentil Soup

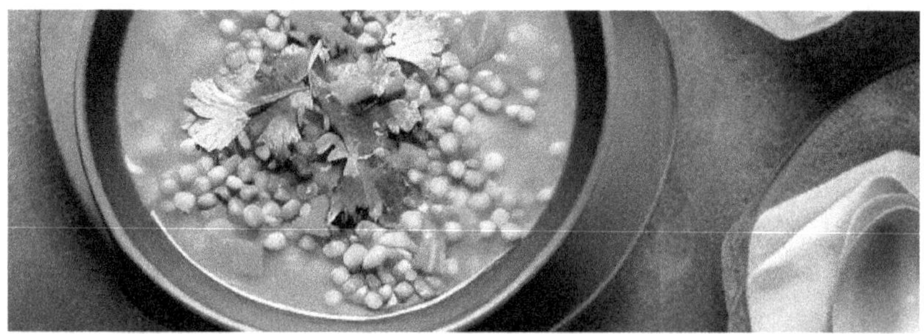

Ingredients:

- 1 tablespoon olive oil
- 1 onion, diced
- 2 carrots, peeled and diced
- 2 celery stalks, diced
- 2 garlic cloves, minced
- 1 cup dry lentils, rinsed
- 6 cups vegetable broth, gluten-free
- 1 teaspoon ground cumin
- 1/2 teaspoon ground coriander
- Salt and pepper to taste
- 1 bay leaf
- 2 tablespoons tomato paste
- Fresh parsley, chopped for garnish

Preparation:

1. Heat olive oil in a large pot over medium heat. Add onion, carrots, celery, and garlic. Cook until vegetables are softened, about 5 minutes.

2. Stir in the rinsed lentils, vegetable broth, cumin, coriander, salt, pepper, bay leaf, and tomato paste.

3. Bring to a boil, then reduce heat to low and simmer, covered, until lentils are tender, about 30 minutes.

4. Remove bay leaf. Use an immersion blender to partially puree the soup for a thicker consistency, if desired.

5. Adjust seasoning to taste. Serve hot, garnished with fresh parsley.

Cooking Time: 45 minutes.

Nutritional Values (per serving):

- Calories: ~230
- Protein: ~14 grams
- Fat: ~4 grams
- Carbohydrates: ~36 grams
- Fiber: ~16 grams
- Sodium: ~700 mg

Rating: ★★★★★

This Lentil Soup is a hearty, nutritious, and comforting meal, filled with flavors that blend perfectly together. It's an excellent source of protein and fiber, making it a satisfying dish that's ideal for anyone seeking a healthful, gluten-free option.

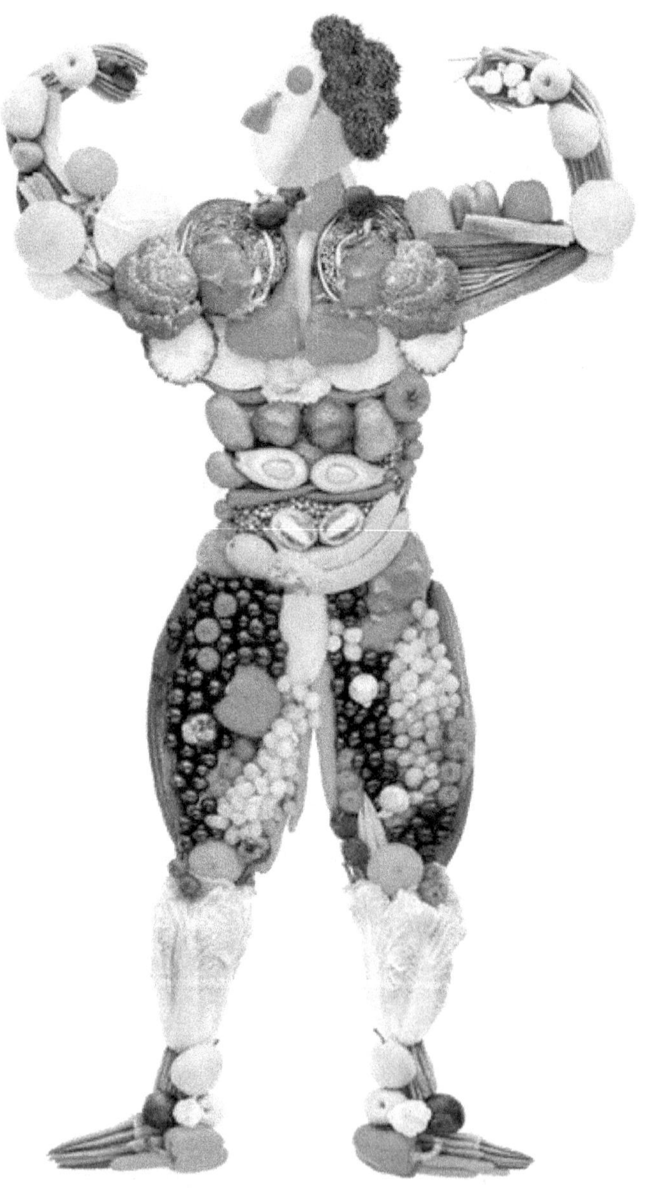

Chapter 5: Salads

Welcome to the Salads section of our cookbook! Dive into a world of fresh, vibrant, and satisfying gluten-free salad recipes that are perfect for any occasion. Whether you're a salad aficionado or just looking to add more greens to your diet, our Salads chapter has something to delight every taste bud. So grab your chopping board, toss together some crisp veggies and tasty dressings, and get ready to enjoy the fresh and delicious flavors of our gluten-free salad recipes.

Kale and Avocado Salad

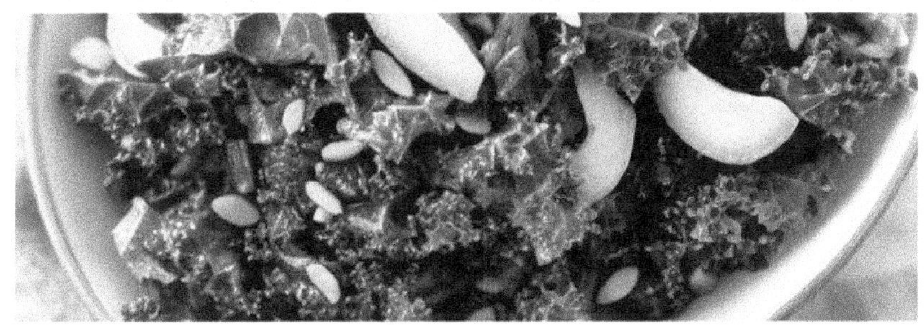

Ingredients:

- 4 cups kale, destemmed and chopped
- 1 ripe avocado, diced
- 1/2 red onion, thinly sliced
- 1/4 cup sliced almonds
- 2 tablespoons lemon juice
- 2 tablespoons olive oil
- Salt and pepper to taste
- Optional: 1/4 cup grated Parmesan cheese

Preparation:

1. In a large bowl, combine the kale, avocado, and red onion.

2. In a small bowl, whisk together the lemon juice, olive oil, salt, and pepper to create the dressing.

3. Pour the dressing over the salad and toss until the kale is well coated and begins to soften.

4. Sprinkle sliced almonds (and Parmesan cheese, if using) over the salad. Toss gently to combine.

5. Serve immediately or let sit for a few minutes to allow flavors to meld.

Cooking Time: 10 minutes.

Nutritional Values (per serving):

- Calories: ~250
- Protein: ~5 grams
- Fat: ~20 grams
- Carbohydrates: ~15 grams
- Fiber: ~7 grams
- Sodium: ~200 mg

Rating: ★★★★☆

This Kale and Avocado Salad is a fresh, nutritious, and vibrant dish. It's rich in healthy fats, vitamins, and fiber. Easy to prepare and customizable with your favorite nuts or cheese, it's a perfect starter or side for any meal, especially for those looking for a healthful, gluten-free option.

Arugula, Pear, and Walnut Salad

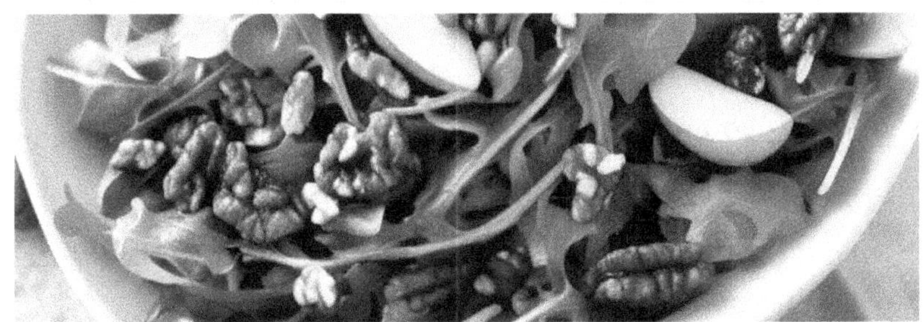

Ingredients:

- 4 cups arugula, washed
- 1 ripe pear, thinly sliced
- 1/2 cup walnuts, toasted
- 1/4 cup crumbled blue cheese (optional)
- 2 tablespoons balsamic vinegar
- 1 tablespoon olive oil
- Salt and pepper to taste

Preparation:

1. In a large salad bowl, combine the arugula, pear slices, and toasted walnuts.

2. If using, sprinkle the crumbled blue cheese over the salad.

3. In a small bowl, whisk together the balsamic vinegar, olive oil, salt, and pepper to create the dressing.

4. Drizzle the dressing over the salad and gently toss to combine, ensuring the ingredients are evenly coated.

5. Serve immediately, adjusting seasoning with salt and pepper if desired.

Cooking Time: About 10 minutes.

Nutritional Values (per serving):

- Calories: ~220
- Protein: ~5 grams
- Fat: ~18 grams
- Carbohydrates: ~12 grams
- Fiber: ~3 grams
- Sodium: ~180 mg

Rating: ★★★★☆

This Arugula, Pear, and Walnut Salad is a delightful blend of peppery, sweet, and nutty flavors, complemented by the tanginess of the balsamic dressing. It's a quick, nutritious, and elegant dish perfect for a light lunch or as a side, offering a wholesome gluten-free option that doesn't compromise on taste.

Mediterranean Quinoa Salad

Ingredients:

- 1 cup quinoa, rinsed
- 2 cups water
- 1 cup cherry tomatoes, halved

- 1 cucumber, diced
- 1/2 red onion, finely chopped
- 1/4 cup Kalamata olives, pitted and sliced
- 1/4 cup feta cheese, crumbled
- 1/4 cup fresh parsley, chopped
- 3 tablespoons olive oil
- 2 tablespoons lemon juice
- Salt and pepper to taste

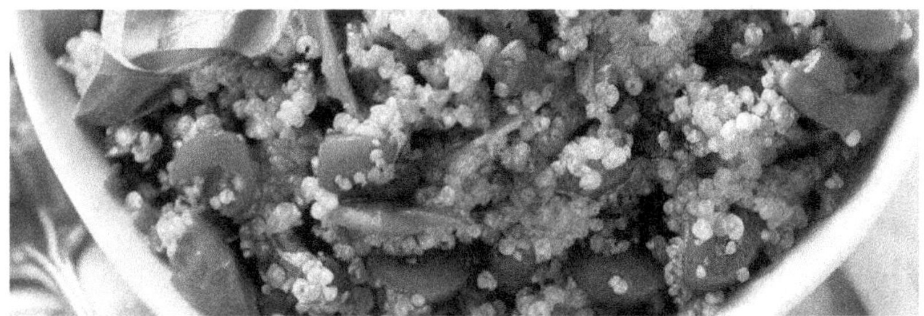

Preparation:

1. In a medium saucepan, bring water to a boil. Add quinoa, reduce heat to low, cover, and simmer for about 15 minutes, or until water is absorbed and quinoa is tender. Allow to cool.

2. In a large bowl, combine cooled quinoa, cherry tomatoes, cucumber, red onion, Kalamata olives, and feta cheese.

3. In a small bowl, whisk together olive oil, lemon juice, salt, and pepper to create the dressing.

4. Pour dressing over the salad and toss to combine. Garnish with fresh parsley.

5. Serve chilled or at room temperature.

Cooking Time: About 25 minutes.

Nutritional Values (per serving):

- Calories: ~260
- Protein: ~8 grams
- Fat: ~14 grams
- Carbohydrates: ~28 grams
- Fiber: ~4 grams
- Sodium: ~300 mg

Rating: ★★★★★

This Mediterranean Quinoa Salad is a vibrant, nutrient-rich dish, perfect for a refreshing meal or side. Its combination of flavors and textures, from the fluffy quinoa to the crisp vegetables and briny olives, makes it a delightful gluten-free option that's both satisfying and healthy.

Spinach and Strawberry Salad

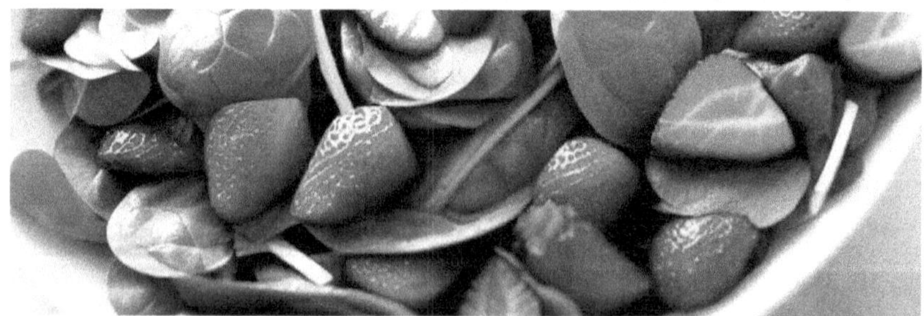

Ingredients:

- 4 cups fresh spinach, washed and dried
- 1 cup strawberries, sliced
- 1/2 cup walnuts, toasted

- 1/4 cup goat cheese, crumbled
- 2 tablespoons balsamic vinegar
- 1 tablespoon olive oil
- 1 teaspoon honey
- Salt and pepper to taste

Preparation:

1. In a large salad bowl, combine the spinach, sliced strawberries, and toasted walnuts.

2. Sprinkle crumbled goat cheese over the top of the salad.

3. In a small bowl, whisk together balsamic vinegar, olive oil, honey, salt, and pepper to create the dressing.

4. Drizzle the dressing over the salad and gently toss to ensure all the ingredients are evenly coated.

5. Serve immediately, enjoying the blend of flavors and textures.

Prep Time: 10 minutes.

Nutritional Values (per serving):

- Calories: ~210
- Protein: ~6 grams
- Fat: ~16 grams
- Carbohydrates: ~12 grams
- Fiber: ~3 grams
- Sodium: ~180 mg

Rating: ★★★★★

This Spinach and Strawberry Salad is a delightful mix of sweet and savory, perfect for a light and healthy meal or side. The creamy goat cheese and crunchy walnuts add texture and richness to the fresh spinach and strawberries, making it a satisfying, gluten-free choice that's both nutritious and flavorful.

Cucumber and Dill Salad

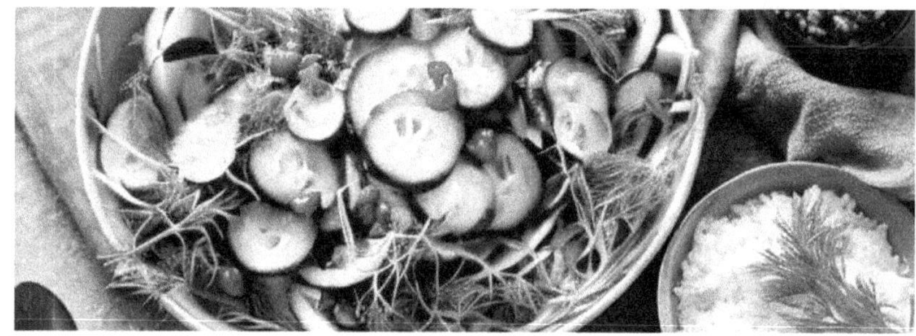

Ingredients:

- 2 large cucumbers, thinly sliced
- 1/4 cup red onion, thinly sliced
- 1/4 cup fresh dill, chopped
- 3 tablespoons white vinegar
- 1 tablespoon olive oil
- 1 teaspoon sugar
- Salt and pepper to taste

Preparation:

1. In a large bowl, combine the thinly sliced cucumbers and red onion.

2. In a small bowl, whisk together the white vinegar, olive oil, sugar, salt, and pepper to create the dressing.

3. Pour the dressing over the cucumber and onion mixture. Add the chopped dill and toss everything together until well combined.

4. Refrigerate for at least 30 minutes before serving to allow flavors to meld.

Cooking Time: About 10 minutes plus chilling time.

Nutritional Values (per serving):

- Calories: ~50
- Protein: ~1 gram
- Fat: ~3.5 grams
- Carbohydrates: ~4 grams
- Fiber: ~1 gram
- Sodium: ~10 mg

Rating: ★★★★☆

This Cucumber and Dill Salad is a refreshing, light side dish perfect for warm days. The crisp cucumbers paired with the tangy dressing and fresh dill create a delightful flavor profile. \

Thai Peanut- Quinoa Salad

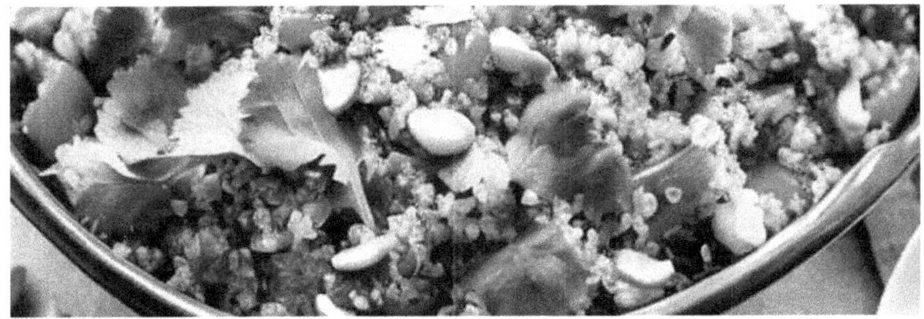

Ingredients:

- 1 cup quinoa, rinsed
- 2 cups water
- 1 red bell pepper, diced
- 1 carrot, julienned
- 1/2 cup red cabbage, shredded
- 1/2 cup cucumber, diced
- 1/4 cup green onions, sliced
- 1/4 cup cilantro, chopped
- **For the Thai Peanut Dressing:**
  - 1/4 cup peanut butter
- 2 tablespoons soy sauce (gluten-free)
- 1 tablespoon honey
- 2 teaspoons fresh ginger, grated
- 1 garlic clove, minced
- 1 tablespoon lime juice
- 1 teaspoon sesame oil
- Water to thin, if needed

Preparation:

1. Cook quinoa in water according to package instructions. Let it cool.

2. In a large bowl, combine the cooled quinoa, red bell pepper, carrot, red cabbage, cucumber, green onions, and cilantro.

3. For the dressing, whisk together peanut butter, soy sauce, honey, ginger, garlic, lime juice, and sesame oil in a small bowl. Add water if needed to achieve desired consistency.

4. Pour the dressing over the salad and toss until everything is well coated.

5. Serve chilled or at room temperature.

Cooking Time: 30 minutes (including quinoa cooking and cooling time).

Nutritional Values (per serving):

- Calories: ~320
- Protein: ~10 grams
- Fat: ~14 grams
- Carbohydrates: ~40 grams
- Fiber: ~5 grams
- Sodium: ~400 mg

Rating: ★★★★★

This Thai Peanut-Quinoa Salad is a vibrant, flavorful dish packed with fresh vegetables and coated in a rich, savory peanut dressing. It offers a delicious balance of textures and tastes, making it a perfect gluten-free meal or side. The combination of healthy ingredients ensures a nutritious and satisfying experience.

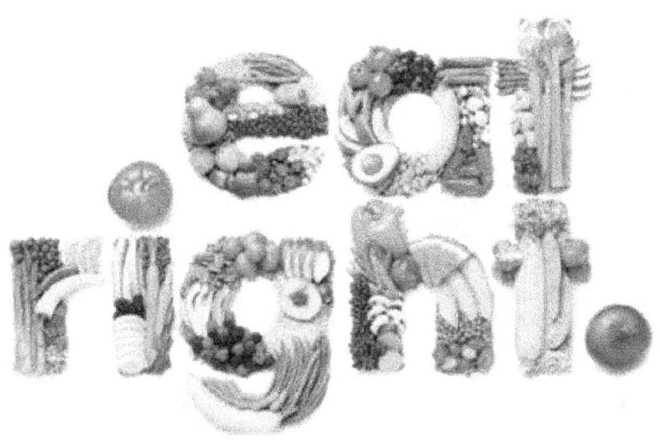

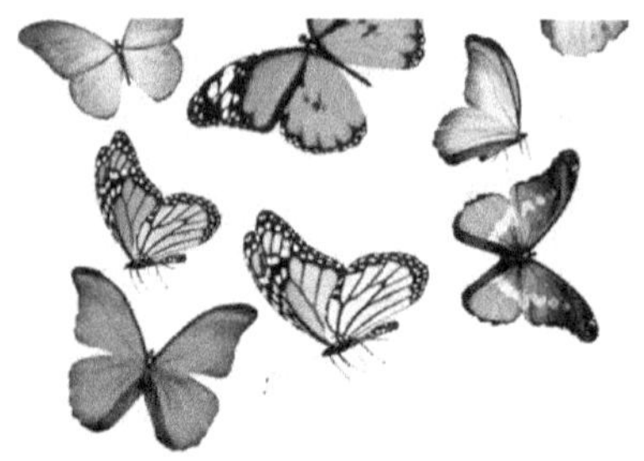

Fuel your body with wholesome, gluten-free delights – from quinoa to kale and everything in between. Every bite nourishes your journey toward reclaiming wellness. Let nutritious foods be your guiding light.

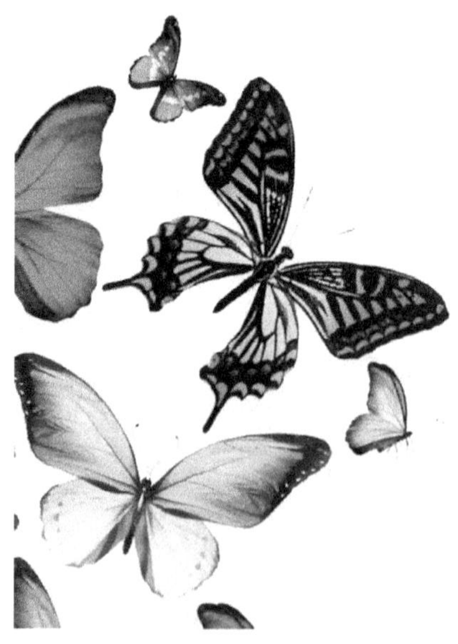

Chapter 6: Beverages

Quench your thirst and tantalize your taste buds with our collection of refreshing gluten-free beverage recipes. From energizing smoothies and creamy milkshakes to soothing herbal teas and invigorating mocktails, we've got a drink for every mood and occasion. Explore unique flavor combinations, experiment with fresh ingredients, and discover your new favorite drink. With easy-to-follow recipes and helpful tips, you'll be mixing up delicious and satisfying beverages in no time. So, grab your blender, cocktail shaker, or tea kettle, and let's raise a glass to the joy of gluten-free drinking!

Green Smoothie

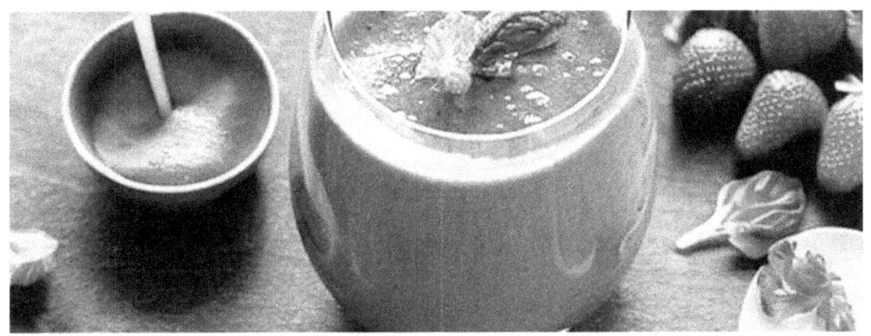

Ingredients:

- 1 cup spinach, fresh
- 1/2 cup kale, destemmed and chopped
- 1 banana, peeled
- 1/2 apple, cored and chopped
- 1 tablespoon chia seeds
- 1 cup almond milk, unsweetened
- Ice cubes (optional)

Preparation:

1. In a blender, combine spinach, kale, banana, apple, chia seeds, and almond milk.

2. Blend on high until smooth. If the smoothie is too thick, add more almond milk to reach desired consistency.

3. Add ice cubes to the blender if you prefer a colder smoothie. Blend again until smooth.

4. Pour into a glass and serve immediately.

Cooking Time: About 5 minutes.

Nutritional Values (per serving):

- Calories: ~180
- Protein: ~3 grams
- Fat: ~4 grams
- Carbohydrates: ~35 grams
- Fiber: ~6 grams
- Sodium: ~80 mg

Rating: ★★★★★

This Green Smoothie is a nutrient-packed, delicious way to start your day or refuel after a workout. Combining leafy greens with fruit and chia seeds, it delivers a powerful mix of vitamins, minerals, and fiber.

Almond Milk Latte

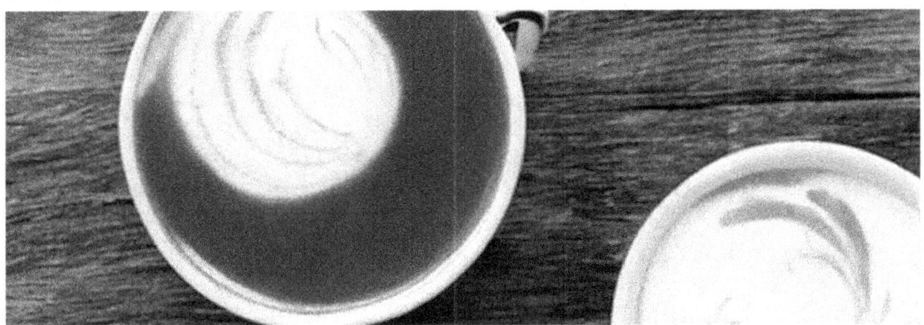

Ingredients:

- 1 cup almond milk, unsweetened
- 2 shots espresso (or 1/2 cup strong brewed coffee)
- 1 teaspoon vanilla extract (optional)
- Cinnamon or cocoa powder for garnish (optional)

Preparation:

1. Heat the almond milk in a saucepan over medium heat until hot but not boiling. Alternatively, use a microwave-safe container and heat in the microwave for about 1 minute.
2. If desired, whisk the hot almond milk vigorously or use a milk frother to create foam.

3. Prepare the espresso or strong brewed coffee.

4. Pour the espresso or coffee into a large mug, add vanilla extract if using, and top with the hot frothed almond milk.

5. Garnish with a sprinkle of cinnamon or cocoa powder if desired.

6. Serve immediately and enjoy.

Cooking Time: About 5 minutes.

Nutritional Values (per serving):

- Calories: ~30 (without espresso/coffee)
- Protein: ~1 gram
- Fat: ~2.5 grams
- Carbohydrates: ~1 gram
- Fiber: ~0 grams
- Sodium: ~180 mg

Rating: ★★★★☆

This Almond Milk Latte is a delicious, dairy-free alternative to traditional lattes, offering a light and nutty flavor. The optional vanilla and garnish of cinnamon or cocoa add a delightful touch.

Mango and Pineapple Smoothie

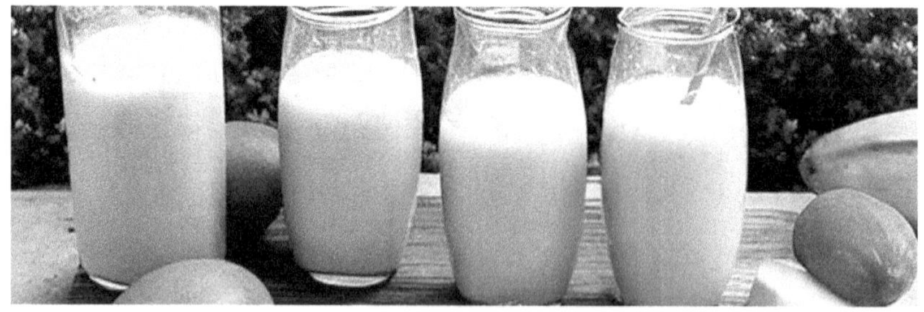

Ingredients:

- 1 cup mango, chopped and frozen
- 1 cup pineapple, chopped and frozen
- 1 banana, peeled
- 1 cup coconut water
- Ice cubes (optional, if you prefer a thicker smoothie)

Preparation:

1. Place the frozen mango, pineapple, banana, and coconut water in a blender.

2. Blend on high until smooth and creamy. Add ice cubes if you're aiming for a thicker consistency, and blend again.

3. Pour the smoothie into glasses and serve immediately.

Cooking Time: 5 minutes.

Nutritional Values (per serving):

- Calories: ~180
- Protein: ~2 grams
- Fat: ~0.5 grams
- Carbohydrates: ~45 grams
- Fiber: ~5 grams
- Sodium: ~40 mg

Rating: ★★★★★

This Mango and Pineapple Smoothie is a tropical delight, bursting with flavors and vitamins. It's an incredibly refreshing choice, perfect for a hot day or as a nutritious snack. With no added sugar and plenty of fiber, it's a healthy, gluten-free option that's as satisfying as it is delicious.

Herbal Tea Infusions

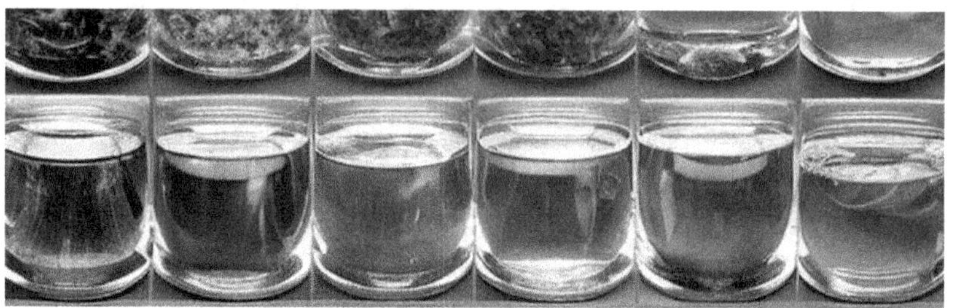

Chamomile Lavender Tea

Ingredients:

- 1 tablespoon dried chamomile flowers
- 1 teaspoon dried lavender buds
- 8 ounces boiling water

Preparation:

1. Combine chamomile flowers and lavender buds in a tea infuser or teapot.

2. Pour boiling water over the herbs and cover.

3. Steep for 5-7 minutes, depending on desired strength.

4. Remove the infuser or strain the tea into a cup.

5. Optional: Sweeten with honey or lemon for extra flavor.

Cooking Time: 10 minutes.

Nutritional Values (per serving):

- Calories: 0 (without honey)
- Protein: 0 grams
- Fat: 0 grams
- Carbohydrates: 0 grams
- Fiber: 0 grams
- Sodium: 0 mg

Rating: ★★★★★

Chamomile Lavender Tea is a soothing, aromatic herbal infusion perfect for relaxing moments or before bedtime. It combines the calming properties of chamomile with the soothing scent of lavender, creating a peaceful escape in every cup.

Mint Ginger Tea

Ingredients:

- 1 tablespoon fresh mint leaves
- 1-inch piece of ginger, thinly sliced
- 8 ounces boiling water

Preparation:

1. Place mint leaves and ginger slices in a mug or teapot.

2. Pour boiling water over the mint and ginger.

3. Cover and steep for 5-10 minutes, depending on how strong you like it.

4. Strain the tea into another cup if needed.

5. Optional: Add honey or lemon to taste.

Cooking Time: 10 minutes.

Nutritional Values (per serving):

- Calories: 0 (without honey)
- Protein: 0 grams
- Fat: 0 grams
- Carbohydrates: 0 grams
- Fiber: 0 grams
- Sodium: 0 mg

Rating: ★★★★★

Mint Ginger Tea is a refreshing and invigorating herbal infusion known for its digestive benefits and energizing properties. The spicy kick of ginger paired with the cooling sensation of mint creates a balanced and flavorful cup, ideal for starting the day or as a pick-me-up in the afternoon. This caffeine-free blend is a healthful choice for anyone seeking a natural boost.

Fruit-Infused Water Variations

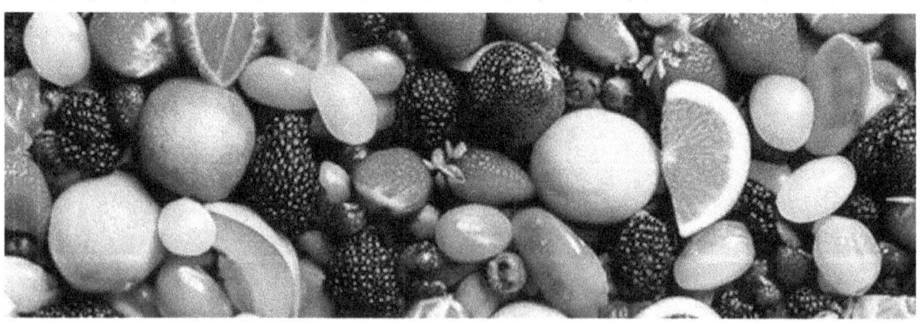

Lemon and Mint Water

Ingredients:

- 1 lemon, thinly sliced
- 10 fresh mint leaves
- 1 liter of water

Preparation:

1. Place lemon slices and mint leaves in a large pitcher.

2. Fill the pitcher with water.

3. Refrigerate for at least 1 hour or overnight to allow flavors to infuse.

4. Serve chilled, adding ice cubes if desired.

Nutritional Values (per serving):

- Calories: 0
- Protein: 0 grams
- Fat: 0 grams
- Carbohydrates: 0 grams (negligible from lemon)
- Fiber: 0 grams
- Sodium: 0 mg

Rating: ★★★★★

Lemon and Mint Water is a refreshing, zesty option perfect for hydration. The lemon adds a nice tang, while mint brings a cooling effect, making it a delightful drink for any time of the day.

Cucumber and Strawberry Water

Ingredients:

- 1/2 cucumber, thinly sliced
- 1/2 cup strawberries, sliced
- 1 liter of water

Preparation:

1. Combine cucumber and strawberry slices in a pitcher.

2. Add water and mix gently.

3. Refrigerate to infuse for 1-2 hours or overnight.

4. Enjoy chilled, adding more fresh slices for garnish if desired.

Nutritional Values (per serving):

- Calories: 0
- Protein: 0 grams
- Fat: 0 grams
- Carbohydrates: 0 grams (negligible from fruit)
- Fiber: 0 grams
- Sodium: 0 mg

Rating: ★★★★★

Cucumber and Strawberry Water offers a unique, subtly sweet flavor with a hint of crisp freshness from the cucumber. It's a visually appealing and hydrating drink that's great for summertime sipping or as a spa-inspired refreshment.

Orange and Blueberry Water

Ingredients:

- 1 orange, thinly sliced
- 1/2 cup blueberries
- 1 liter of water

Preparation:

1. Add orange slices and blueberries to a large pitcher.

2. Pour water over the fruits.

3. Refrigerate for a few hours or overnight to let the flavors meld.

4. Serve cold, optionally with ice.

Nutritional Values (per serving):

- Calories: 0
- Protein: 0 grams
- Fat: 0 grams
- Carbohydrates: 0 grams (negligible from fruits)
- Fiber: 0 grams
- Sodium: 0 mg

Rating: ★★★★★

Orange and Blueberry Water is a sweet and tangy infusion, bursting with antioxidants and vitamin C. The combination of citrus and berries creates a vibrant, flavorful drink that's as nutritious as it is delicious, perfect for boosting hydration and refreshing the palate.

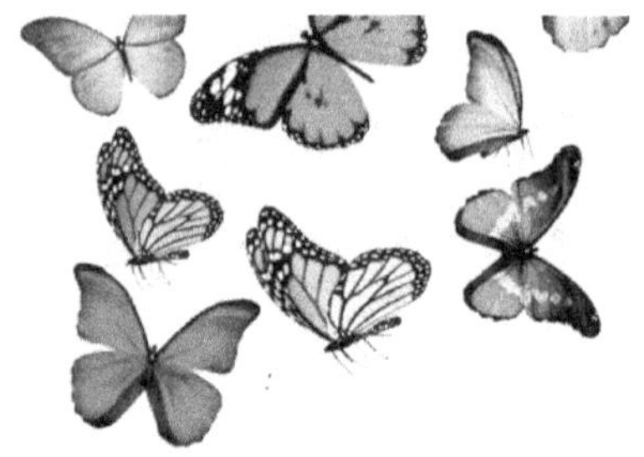

Your plate is your canvas for wellness. Load it with wholesome, gluten-free treasures that nourish your body and soul. With each meal, you rewrite your story of strength and resilience against celiac disease.

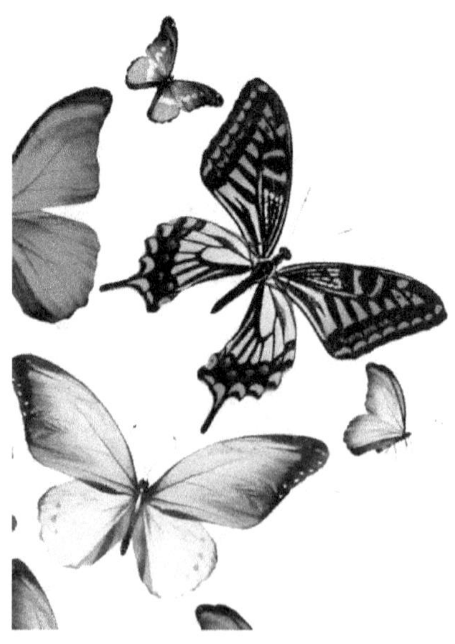

Chapter 7: Meat and Poultry

Prepare to indulge in a delectable selection of gluten-free dishes with substantial meats and poultry. From mouthwatering roasts and fragrant marinades to sizzling stir-fries and cozy casseroles, we've collected a collection of delectable dishes to satiate your meat-loving desires.

Herb-Crusted Chicken Breast

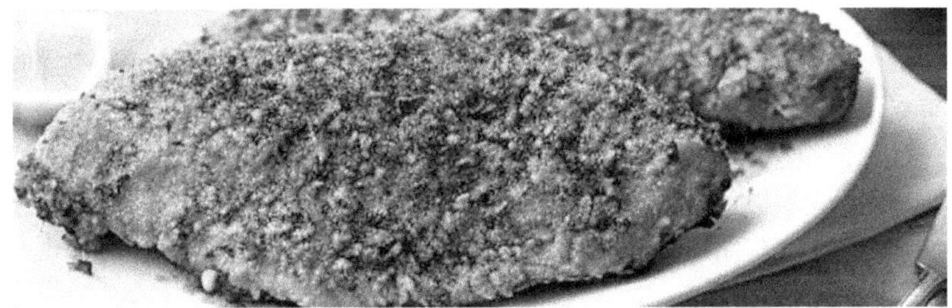

Ingredients:

- 2 boneless, skinless chicken breasts
- 1 tablespoon olive oil
- 1/2 cup gluten-free breadcrumbs

- 2 tablespoons fresh parsley, chopped
- 1 teaspoon fresh thyme, chopped
- 1 teaspoon fresh rosemary, chopped
- Salt and pepper to taste
- 1 egg, beaten

Preparation:

1. Preheat the oven to 375°F (190°C).

2. Season the chicken breasts with salt and pepper.

3. Mix the breadcrumbs, parsley, thyme, and rosemary in a shallow dish.

4. Dip each chicken breast in the beaten egg, then coat thoroughly with the breadcrumb mixture.

5. Heat olive oil in a skillet over medium heat. Sear the chicken for 2 minutes on each side, or until golden.

6. Transfer the chicken to a baking dish and bake in the oven for 20-25 minutes, or until the chicken is cooked through and no longer pink inside.

7. Serve hot, garnished with additional herbs if desired.

Cooking Time: About 30 minutes.

Nutritional Values (per serving):

- Calories: ~300
- Protein: ~26 grams

- Fat: ~12 grams
- Carbohydrates: ~18 grams
- Fiber: ~1 gram
- Sodium: ~200 mg

Rating: ★★★★☆

This Herb-Crusted Chicken Breast is a flavorful, juicy dish with a delightful crispy coating. The blend of fresh herbs brings out a fragrant and savory taste that complements the tender chicken perfectly. It's a simple yet delicious option for a nutritious meal, suitable for those following a gluten-free diet.

Beef Stir-Fry with Vegetables

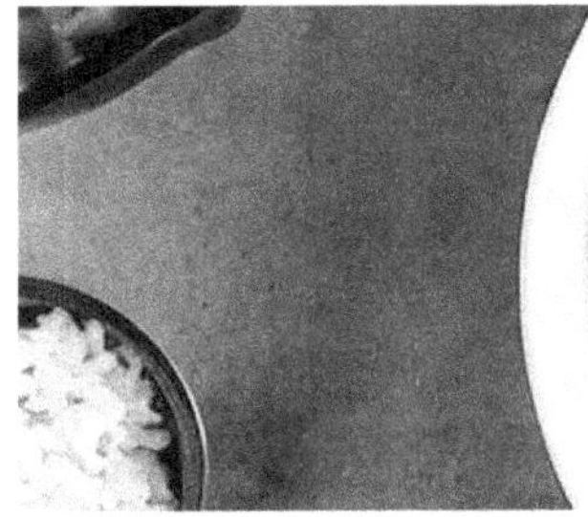
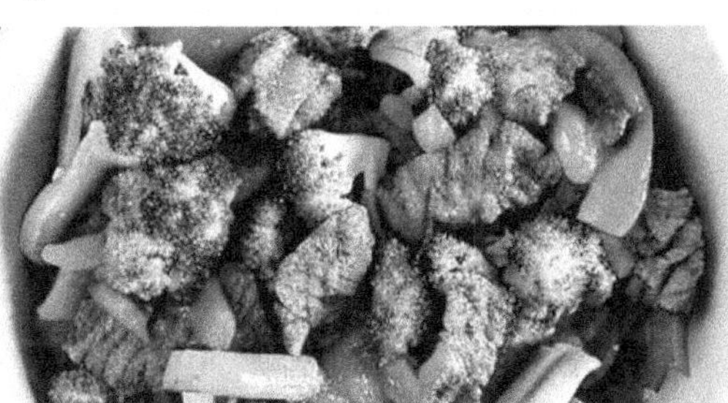

Ingredients:

- 1 pound beef sirloin, thinly sliced
- 2 tablespoons soy sauce (gluten-free)
- 1 tablespoon sesame oil
- 1 tablespoon olive oil
- 2 cups mixed vegetables (e.g., bell peppers, broccoli, snap peas, carrots)
- 1 onion, sliced
- 2 garlic cloves, minced
- 1 teaspoon ginger, grated

- Salt and pepper to taste

Preparation:

1. In a bowl, marinate the beef slices in soy sauce and sesame oil for at least 15 minutes.

2. Heat olive oil in a large pan or wok over medium-high heat.

3. Add the marinated beef slices and cook for 2-3 minutes until browned. Remove and set aside.

4. In the same pan, add onion, garlic, and ginger. Sauté for 2 minutes until fragrant.

5. Add the mixed vegetables and cook for 5-7 minutes, stirring frequently, until they are just tender but still crisp.

6. Return the beef to the pan. Stir well to combine and cook for another 2 minutes.

7. Season with salt and pepper to taste. Serve hot.

Cooking Time: About 30 minutes.

Nutritional Values (per serving):

- Calories: ~300
- Protein: ~25 grams
- Fat: ~15 grams
- Carbohydrates: ~15 grams
- Fiber: ~3 grams
- Sodium: ~700 mg

Rating: ★★★★☆

This Beef Stir-Fry with Vegetables is a vibrant, flavorful dish that combines tender slices of beef with a colorful mix of vegetables, all seasoned with a savory blend of soy sauce, sesame oil, and fresh ginger. It's a quick and easy meal, perfect for a busy weeknight, and a great way to incorporate a variety of vegetables into your diet.

Lemon-Garlic Roasted Turkey

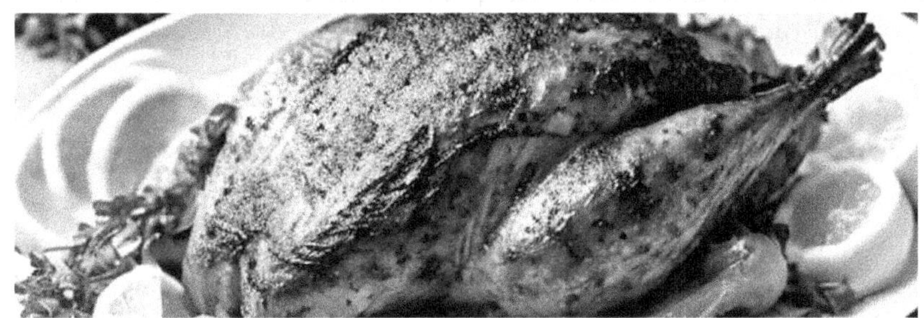

Ingredients:

- 1 whole turkey (about 12 pounds), thawed
- 4 lemons, halved
- 1 head of garlic, halved horizontally
- 1/4 cup olive oil
- 2 tablespoons fresh thyme, chopped
- Salt and pepper to taste
- 1 onion, quartered
- 4 cups low-sodium chicken broth (for the roasting pan)

Preparation:

1. Preheat your oven to 325°F (165°C).

2. Pat the turkey dry with paper towels. Season the cavity with salt and pepper. Stuff it with lemon halves, garlic halves, and onion quarters.

3. Rub the outside of the turkey with olive oil, then season it generously with salt, pepper, and thyme.

4. Place the turkey breast-side up on a rack in a roasting pan. Pour chicken broth into the bottom of the pan.

5. Roast the turkey in the preheated oven, basting occasionally with the pan juices, for about 3 to 3 1/2 hours, or until an internal thermometer inserted into the thickest part of the thigh reads 165°F (74°C).

6. Let the turkey rest for at least 20 minutes before carving. Serve with the pan juices.

Cooking Time: About 3.5 hours, plus resting time.

Nutritional Values (per serving):

- Calories: ~450
- Protein: ~70 grams
- Fat: ~20 grams
- Carbohydrates: ~5 grams
- Fiber: ~1 gram
- Sodium: ~300 mg

Rating: ★★★★★

This Lemon-Garlic Roasted Turkey is a succulent, flavorful centerpiece perfect for any special occasion. The lemon and garlic infuse the meat with a bright, aromatic flavor, while the olive oil and thyme create a deliciously crispy skin. It's a simple yet elegant dish that's sure to impress your guests, making it a top choice for a festive meal.

Pork Chops with Apple Cider Vinegar Sauce

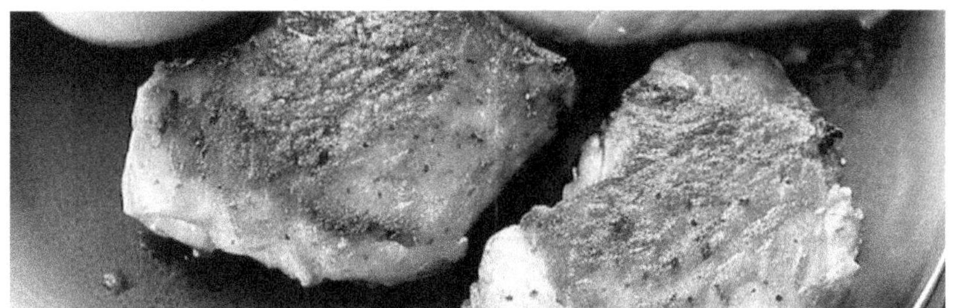

Ingredients:

- 4 pork chops
- 1/4 cup apple cider vinegar
- 2 tablespoons olive oil
- 2 cloves garlic, minced
- 1 teaspoon dried thyme
- Salt and pepper to taste
- Optional: chopped fresh parsley for garnish

Preparation:

1. Season the pork chops with salt, pepper, and dried thyme on both sides.
2. In a skillet, heat olive oil over medium-high heat. Add the pork chops and cook for 4-5 minutes on each side, or until browned and cooked through. Remove from skillet and set aside.

3. In the same skillet, add minced garlic and cook for about 1 minute until fragrant.

4. Stir in apple cider vinegar, scraping up any browned bits from the bottom of the skillet. Allow the vinegar to reduce slightly, about 2-3 minutes.

5. Return the pork chops to the skillet, coating them with the apple cider vinegar sauce. Cook for an additional 2 minutes, until heated through.

6. Serve the pork chops drizzled with the apple cider vinegar sauce, and garnish with chopped fresh parsley if desired.

Cooking Time: Approximately 20 minutes.

Nutritional Values (per serving):

- Calories: ~300
- Protein: ~30 grams
- Fat: ~18 grams
- Carbohydrates: ~2 grams
- Fiber: ~0 grams

Rating: ★★★★☆

These Pork Chops with Apple Cider Vinegar Sauce are a savory and tangy delight, perfect for a quick and flavorful dinner. The apple cider vinegar adds a refreshing zing to the dish, while the pork chops remain juicy and tender. It's a simple yet impressive meal that's sure to earn rave reviews at the table.

Grilled Lamb with Mint Pesto

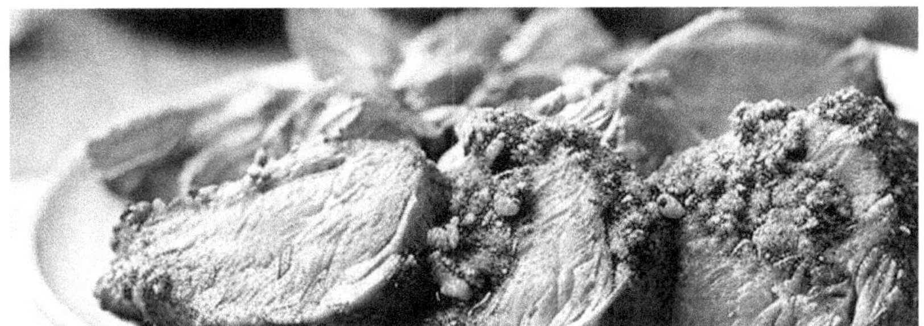

Ingredients:

- 2 pounds lamb chops
- Salt and pepper to taste
- Olive oil for grilling
- **For the Mint Pesto:**
    - 1 cup fresh mint leaves
    - 1/2 cup fresh parsley leaves
- 1/4 cup grated Parmesan cheese
- 1/4 cup pine nuts
- 2 garlic cloves
- 1/2 cup olive oil
- Salt and pepper to taste

Preparation:

1. Season lamb chops with salt and pepper, lightly coating them with olive oil.

2. Preheat the grill to medium-high heat.

3. Grill the lamb chops for about 3-4 minutes per side for medium-rare, or until they reach your desired level of doneness.

4. For the mint pesto, combine mint leaves, parsley, Parmesan cheese, pine nuts, and garlic in a food processor. Pulse until coarsely chopped.

5. While the processor is running, gradually add 1/2 cup olive oil until the mixture is smooth. Season with salt and pepper.

6. Serve the grilled lamb chops with a dollop of mint pesto on top.

Cooking Time: About 20 minutes.

Nutritional Values (per serving):

- Calories: ~600
- Protein: ~35 grams
- Fat: ~50 grams
- Carbohydrates: ~3 grams
- Fiber: ~1 gram
- Sodium: ~200 mg

Rating: ★★★★★

This Grilled Lamb with Mint Pesto is a luxurious, flavorful dish that pairs the rich taste of lamb with the fresh, vibrant flavors of mint and parsley. The homemade pesto adds a creamy texture and a burst of herbal goodness, elevating the lamb chops to a gourmet level. Perfect for a special occasion or a sophisticated dinner, it's sure to delight any palate.

Chapter 8: Seafoods and Fish

Dive into a world of oceanic delights with our collection of delectable gluten-free seafood and fish recipes. From succulent shrimp and tender scallops to flaky salmon and meaty tuna, we've got something to satisfy every seafood lover's palate. With easy-to-follow instructions and helpful tips, you'll be cooking up restaurant-quality seafood dishes right in your own kitchen. So cast your culinary net wide and get ready to reel in the deliciousness with our gluten-free seafood and fish recipes.

Grilled Shrimp Skewers

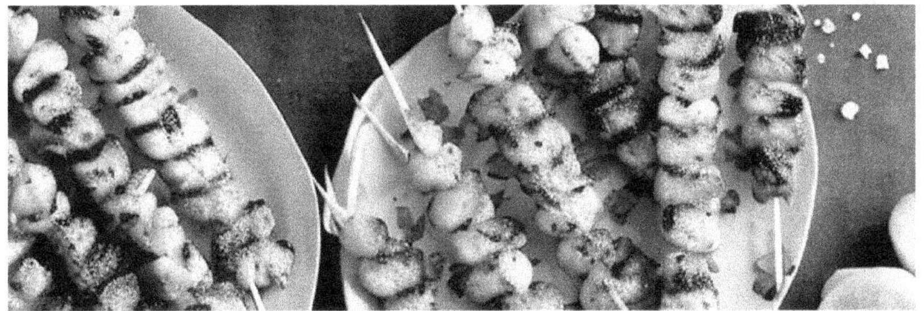

Ingredients:

- 1-pound large shrimp, peeled and deveined
- 2 tablespoons olive oil
- 1 lemon, zest and juice
- 2 garlic cloves, minced
- 1 teaspoon paprika
- Salt and pepper to taste
- Wooden or metal skewers

Preparation:

1. In a bowl, combine olive oil, lemon zest, lemon juice, minced garlic, paprika, salt, and pepper.

2. Add the shrimp to the marinade and toss to coat evenly. Let marinate for 15-30 minutes in the refrigerator.

3. Preheat the grill to medium-high heat.

4. Thread the marinated shrimp onto skewers.

5. Grill the shrimp skewers for 2-3 minutes on each side, or until the shrimp are opaque and cooked through.

6. Serve immediately, optionally with additional lemon wedges on the side.

Cooking Time: About 10 minutes, plus marinating time.

Nutritional Values (per serving):

- Calories: ~220
- Protein: ~24 grams
- Fat: ~12 grams
- Carbohydrates: ~3 grams
- Fiber: ~0 grams
- Sodium: ~200 mg

Rating: ★★★★★

These Grilled Shrimp Skewers are a quick, easy, and incredibly flavorful dish, perfect for any occasion. The combination of lemon, garlic, and paprika provides a vibrant and zesty flavor that complements the natural sweetness of the shrimp. Whether it's a casual barbecue or an elegant dinner, these skewers are sure to impress with their delicious taste and eye-catching presentation.

Pan-Seared Scallops

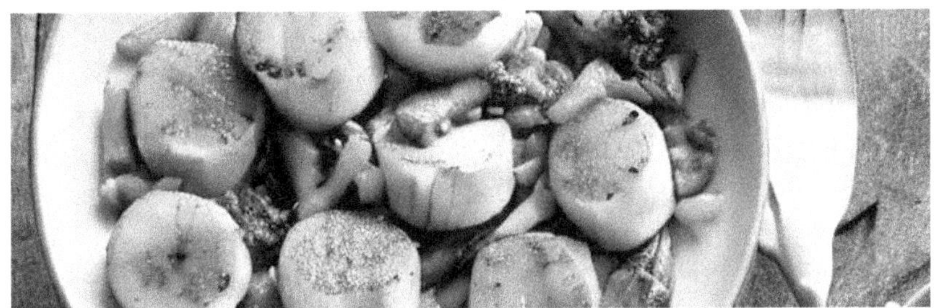

Ingredients:

- 1 pound sea scallops, patted dry
- 2 tablespoons olive oil
- Salt and pepper to taste
- 1 tablespoon unsalted butter
- Lemon wedges, for serving

Preparation:

1. Season the scallops with salt and pepper.

2. Heat olive oil in a large skillet over high heat until hot but not smoking.

3. Add the scallops to the skillet in a single layer, making sure they are not touching. Sear for about 1-2 minutes on each side, until a golden crust forms and they are just cooked through.

4. Add butter to the skillet in the last minute of cooking, spooning it over the scallops.

5. Remove from heat and serve immediately with lemon wedges on the side.

Cooking Time: About 5 minutes.

Nutritional Values (per serving):

- Calories: ~200
- Protein: ~20 grams
- Fat: ~12 grams
- Carbohydrates: ~5 grams
- Fiber: ~0 grams
- Sodium: ~200 mg

Rating: ★★★★★

Pan-Seared Scallops are a simple yet elegant dish that boasts a delicate texture and rich flavor. Perfectly seared on the outside and tender on the inside, these scallops make for a quick, gourmet meal that's sure to impress. The addition of butter enhances their natural sweetness, while a squeeze of lemon adds just the right amount of zesty brightness.

Baked Cod with Lemon and Dill

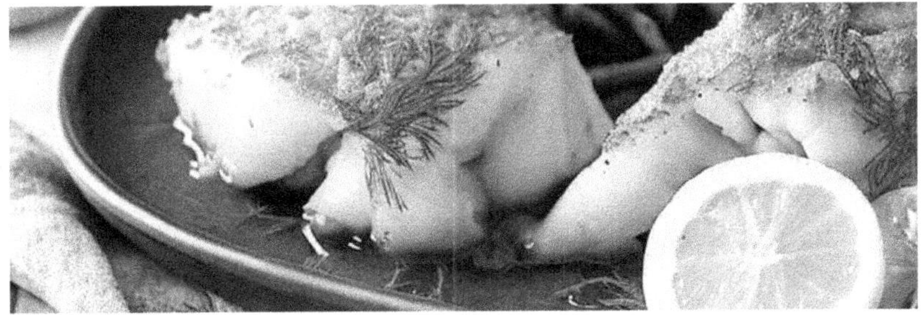

Ingredients:

- 4 cod fillets (about 6 ounces each)
- 2 tablespoons olive oil
- 1 lemon, thinly sliced
- 2 teaspoons fresh dill, chopped
- Salt and pepper to taste

Preparation:

1. Preheat oven to 400°F (200°C).

2. Place cod fillets in a baking dish. Drizzle with olive oil and season with salt and pepper.

3. Top each fillet with lemon slices and sprinkle with dill.

4. Bake in the preheated oven for 12-15 minutes, or until the fish flakes easily with a fork.

5. Serve immediately, garnished with additional dill and lemon wedges if desired.

Cooking Time: About 15 minutes.

Nutritional Values (per serving):

- Calories: ~200
- Protein: ~22 grams
- Fat: ~10 grams
- Carbohydrates: ~2 grams
- Fiber: ~0 grams
- Sodium: ~75 mg

Rating: ★★★★★

Baked Cod with Lemon and Dill is a light, flavorful dish that embodies simplicity and elegance. The subtle flavors of lemon and dill complement the delicate texture of the cod beautifully, making it a perfect choice for a healthy, satisfying meal. Quick and easy to prepare, it's ideal for a weeknight dinner or a special occasion.

Salmon Cakes

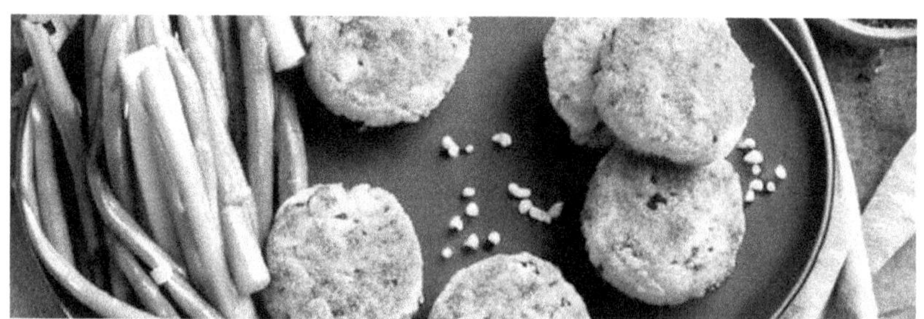

Ingredients:

- 1-pound canned salmon, drained and flaked
- 1/2 cup breadcrumbs (gluten-free for a GF option)
- 2 green onions, finely chopped
- 2 eggs, beaten
- 2 tablespoons mayonnaise
- 1 teaspoon Dijon mustard

- 1/2 teaspoon paprika
- Salt and pepper to taste
- 2 tablespoons olive oil for frying

Preparation:

1. In a large bowl, combine salmon, breadcrumbs, green onions, eggs, mayonnaise, Dijon mustard, paprika, salt, and pepper. Mix well.

2. Form the mixture into patties, about 3-4 inches in diameter.

3. Heat olive oil in a large skillet over medium heat.

4. Fry the salmon cakes for 3-4 minutes on each side, or until golden brown and crispy.

5. Serve hot, optionally with a side of lemon wedges or tartar sauce.

Cooking Time: About 20 minutes.

Nutritional Values (per serving):

- Calories: ~250
- Protein: ~23 grams
- Fat: ~15 grams
- Carbohydrates: ~7 grams
- Fiber: ~1 gram
- Sodium: ~400 mg

Rating: ★★★★☆

Salmon Cakes are a delightful and nutritious dish, featuring the rich flavors of salmon mixed with a light, crispy breadcrumb coating. They're an excellent source of protein and omega-3 fatty acids, making them a healthy choice for any meal. Easy to prepare and versatile, these cakes can be served as a main dish, appetizer, or even tucked into sandwiches for a tasty twist.

Tuna Salad Stuffed Avocados

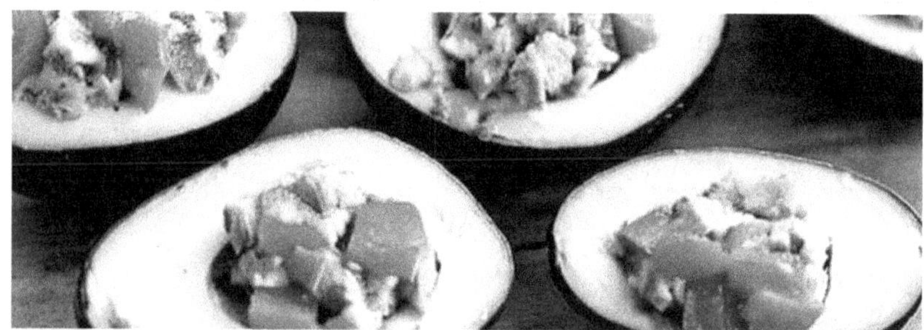

Ingredients:

- 2 ripe avocados, halved and pitted
- 1 can (5 ounces) tuna, drained
- 1/4 cup mayonnaise
- 1/4 cup red onion, finely chopped
- 2 tablespoons celery, finely chopped
- 1 tablespoon lemon juice
- Salt and pepper to taste
- Fresh dill for garnish (optional)

Preparation:

1. In a bowl, mix together tuna, mayonnaise, red onion, celery, and lemon juice. Season with salt and pepper to taste.

2. Scoop out some of the avocado flesh to create more space, if desired. Chop the removed avocado and stir it into the tuna mixture.

3. Fill each avocado half with the tuna salad mixture.

4. Garnish with fresh dill before serving, if using.

Cooking Time: About 10 minutes.

Nutritional Values (per serving):

- Calories: ~300
- Protein: ~15 grams
- Fat: ~25 grams
- Carbohydrates: ~9 grams
- Fiber: ~7 grams
- Sodium: ~200 mg

Rating: ★★★★★

Tuna Salad Stuffed Avocados offer a refreshing, nutritious, and filling dish, combining the creamy texture of avocado with the savory taste of tuna salad. This no-cook recipe is perfect for a quick lunch, snack, or a healthy appetizer, providing a good balance of protein, healthy fats, and fiber. Its simplicity and deliciousness make it a crowd-pleaser.

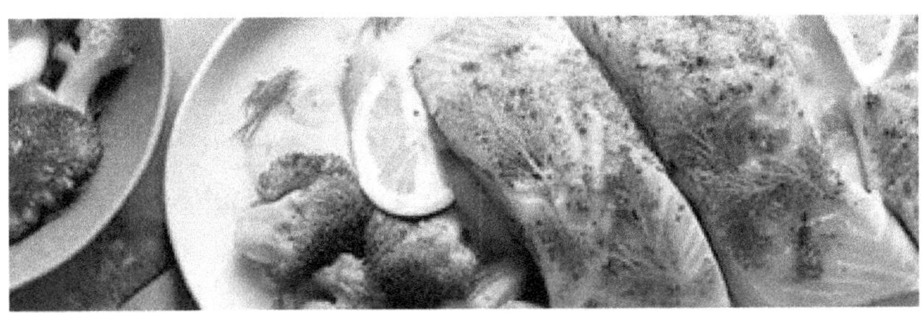

Additional Topics

Navigating Eating Out and Social Events

Navigating eating out and attending social events can be challenging for those on a gluten-free diet due to celiac disease. However, with careful planning and communication, it's possible to enjoy dining out and socializing without compromising your health or dietary restrictions

1. **Research Restaurants in Advance**
   - Look for places that provide a gluten-free menu or are recognized to accommodate particular dietary demands. Many places now serve great gluten-free options.
   - Check internet reviews and menus for gluten-free options and cooking standards to prevent cross-contamination.

2. **Communicate your needs.**
   - Clearly communicate dietary restrictions to the service or chef. Don't be afraid to ask questions about how foods are prepared.

- Be detailed and clear about the severity of your disease. For example, explain that you have celiac disease and cannot consume any gluten, even in small amounts.

3. **Choose Wisely.**

- Choose naturally gluten-free dishes to reduce the danger of cross-contamination. Grilled meats, salads (without croutons), and steamed veggies are generally considered safer options.

- Only eat fried meals at restaurants with specialized gluten-free fryers to prevent cross-contamination.

4. **Be Prepared**

- Pack gluten-free snacks in case of restricted food alternatives during social events.

- Bring your own gluten-free condiments, salad dressings, or bread if the restaurant or event does not provide them.

5. **Advocate for yourself.**

- Be open about your needs. Your health is vital, and most places will accommodate you.

- If you are uncomfortable with the existing selections, you can decline and suggest an alternate venue or bring your own meal if the host allows.

6. **Socialize Beyond Food**

- Prioritize the social component of events over the food. Enjoy both the company and the experience.

- Promote gluten-free eating to friends and family by hosting parties with customizable food options.

Implementing these strategies:

Eating out and attending social events with celiac disease can still be pleasurable. With a little planning and awareness, you can handle these situations comfortably and safely, allowing you to maintain a gluten-free diet while still enjoying the delights of dining and socializing.

Gluten-Free Snacks and Quick Eats

Incorporating gluten-free snacks and quick eats into your diet can be both satisfying and simple.:

1. Fresh Fruits and Vegetables

- Apples, bananas, carrots, and celery sticks are nutritious and naturally gluten-free. Pair with peanut butter or almond butter for added protein.

2. Cheese and Crackers

- Gluten-free crackers paired with cheese make for a satisfying snack. Many brands offer delicious gluten-free options that taste just as good as their gluten-containing counterparts.

3. Yogurt and Granola

- **Plain Greek yogurt** topped with gluten-free granola and fresh berries. Look for granolas that are certified gluten-free to avoid cross-contamination.

4. Nuts and Seeds

- Almonds, walnuts, pumpkin seeds, and sunflower seeds are great for snacking. They're packed with healthy fats, proteins, and fibers. Ensure they are not processed or flavored with gluten-containing ingredients.

5. Popcorn

- Air-popped popcorn is a light and gluten-free snack. Avoid pre-packaged microwave popcorn and make your own to ensure it's gluten-free. Season with your favorite herbs and spices.

6. Rice Cakes and Toppings

- Rice cakes can be topped with avocado, tomato, and salt for a quick and easy snack. They also pair well with hummus or cream cheese and smoked salmon.

7. Homemade Smoothies

- Blend your favorite fruits, vegetables, and a protein source like Greek yogurt or a gluten-free protein powder. Smoothies are a great way to get a nutritious snack or meal on the go.

8. Gluten-Free Bars

- Gluten-free protein or snack bars can be a convenient option. Read labels carefully to ensure they are safe and free from cross-contamination.

9. Hard-Boiled Eggs

- Eggs are an excellent source of protein and very versatile. Hard-boiled eggs make a great grab-and-go snack.

10. Hummus and Veggies

- Hummus is a delicious and healthy dip made from chickpeas. Enjoy it with sliced bell peppers, cucumbers, or carrot sticks.

These gluten-free snacks and quick eats are not only safe for you but also nutritious and delicious options for anyone looking to reduce gluten in their diet. Always remember to check labels for certification and allergen information to ensure products are truly gluten-free.

Understanding Food Labels and Cross-Contamination

Understanding food labels and cross-contamination is crucial for managing a gluten-free diet, especially for individuals with celiac disease. Here's a guide to help navigate these challenges:

Understanding Food Labels:

- **Look for Gluten-Free Certification:** Many products now carry a gluten-free certification or statement. These products have been tested to meet strict gluten-free standards.

- **Read Ingredients Carefully:** Ingredients derived from wheat, barley, rye, and oats (unless labeled gluten-free) contain gluten. Watch out for hidden sources of gluten such as malt, brewer's yeast, and wheat starch.

- **Beware of "May Contain" Statements:** These warnings indicate potential cross-contamination with gluten-containing grains. If you have celiac disease, it's best to avoid these products.

Identifying Cross-Contamination:

- **In the Kitchen:** Use separate utensils, cutting boards, and cookware for gluten-free foods. A toaster used for gluten-containing bread, for example, can contaminate gluten-free bread.

- **When Dining Out:** Inform your server or chef about your gluten sensitivity or celiac disease to ensure they take precautions against cross-contamination.

- **With Packaged Foods:** Facilities that process both gluten-free and gluten-containing products may have a risk of cross-contamination, even if measures are taken to prevent it.

Tips for Avoiding Cross-Contamination:

- **Educate Your Household:** If you live with others who consume gluten, educate them about cross-contamination and establish kitchen rules to keep gluten-free foods safe.

- **Dedicate Gluten-Free Spaces:** Consider having a dedicated gluten-free section in your kitchen, including specific appliances like a gluten-free toaster.

- **Use Labels:** Labeling gluten-free foods and storage containers can help everyone in your household identify safe foods and reduce the risk of accidental cross-contamination.

Traveling and Social Events:

- **Bring Your Own Food:** When attending social events or traveling, bringing your own gluten-free snacks or meals can ensure you have safe options.

- **Communicate Your Needs:** Don't hesitate to communicate your dietary restrictions when attending events or eating at someone else's home. Most hosts are willing to accommodate.

Building a Gluten-Free Pantry: Essentials and Staples

Building a gluten-free pantry is essential for anyone following a gluten-free diet, whether due to celiac disease, gluten sensitivity, or personal preference. Stocking up on gluten-free essentials and staples ensures you always have safe and delicious options on hand. Here's a list to get you started:

Gluten-Free Grains and Flours:

- Brown rice
- Quinoa
- Buckwheat
- Cornmeal
- Oats labeled gluten-free
- Almond flour
- Coconut flour
- Gluten-free all-purpose flour blend
- Baking Ingredients:
- Gluten-free baking powder
- Baking soda
- Xanthan gum or guar gum (for binding in gluten-free baking)
- Vanilla extract
- Cocoa powder
- Honey or maple syrup
- Coconut sugar or other alternative sweeteners

Condiments and Sauces:

- Gluten-free soy sauce or tamari
- Gluten-free Worcestershire sauce
- Rice vinegar

- Balsamic vinegar

- Mustard

- Mayonnaise

- Tomato sauce and paste

- Salsa

Oils and Vinegars:

- Olive oil

- Coconut oil

- Avocado oil

- Apple cider vinegar

- White vinegar

Canned and Jarred Goods:

- Canned beans (e.g., black beans, chickpeas)

- Canned tomatoes

- Coconut milk

- Chicken or vegetable broth

- Nut butters (e.g., peanut butter, almond butter)

- Olives

- Pickles

Snacks and Quick Eats:

- Nuts and seeds

- Dried fruits

- Rice cakes

- Popcorn kernels

- Gluten-free granola bars

- Rice crackers

Miscellaneous:

- Gluten-free pasta

- Gluten-free oats

- Gluten-free breadcrumbs

- Dried herbs and spices

- Nutritional yeast

- Gluten-free baking mixes (e.g., pancake mix, brownie mix)

Experiment with different ingredients and recipes to discover new favorites and enjoy the benefits of a gluten-free lifestyle.

Scan to Gain access to more cookbooks from Joan

For further Questions and advice reach out on

joanmilonehelpdesk@gmail.com

Thank You

I'm writing this with a heart full of gratitude for your kind words and the time you took to read my book, knowing that my words have resonated with you is a reward beyond measure. Thank you again for your appreciation and for being a part of this literary journey.

Warmly,

Joan

>>>
30 Days
Meal
Planner

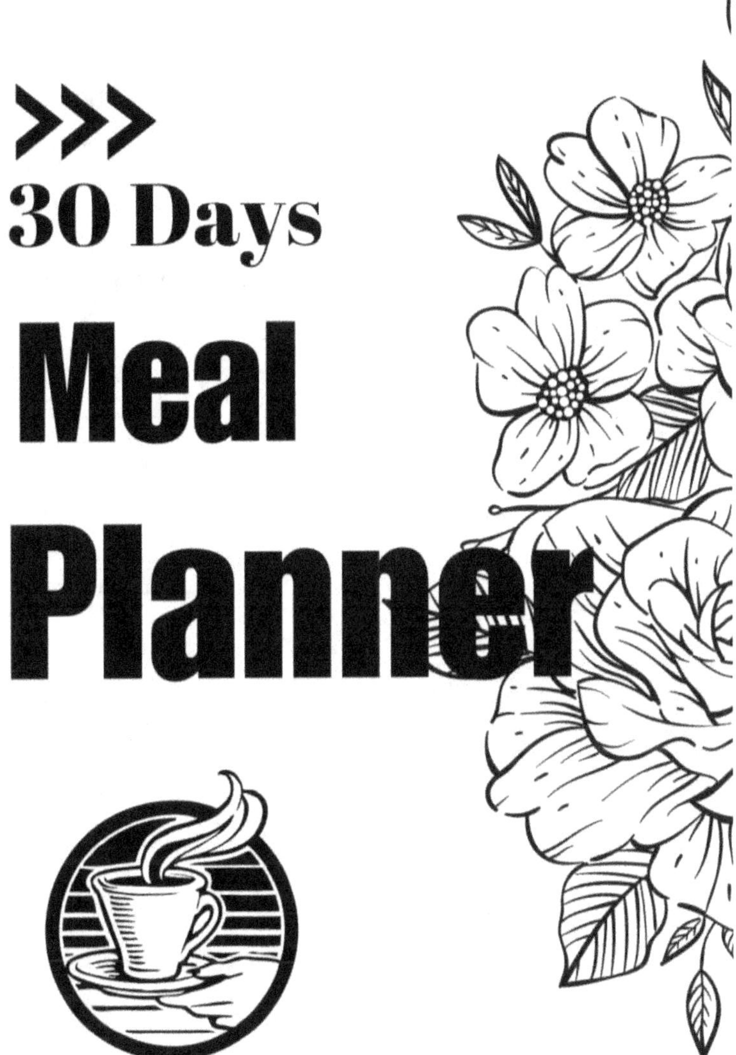

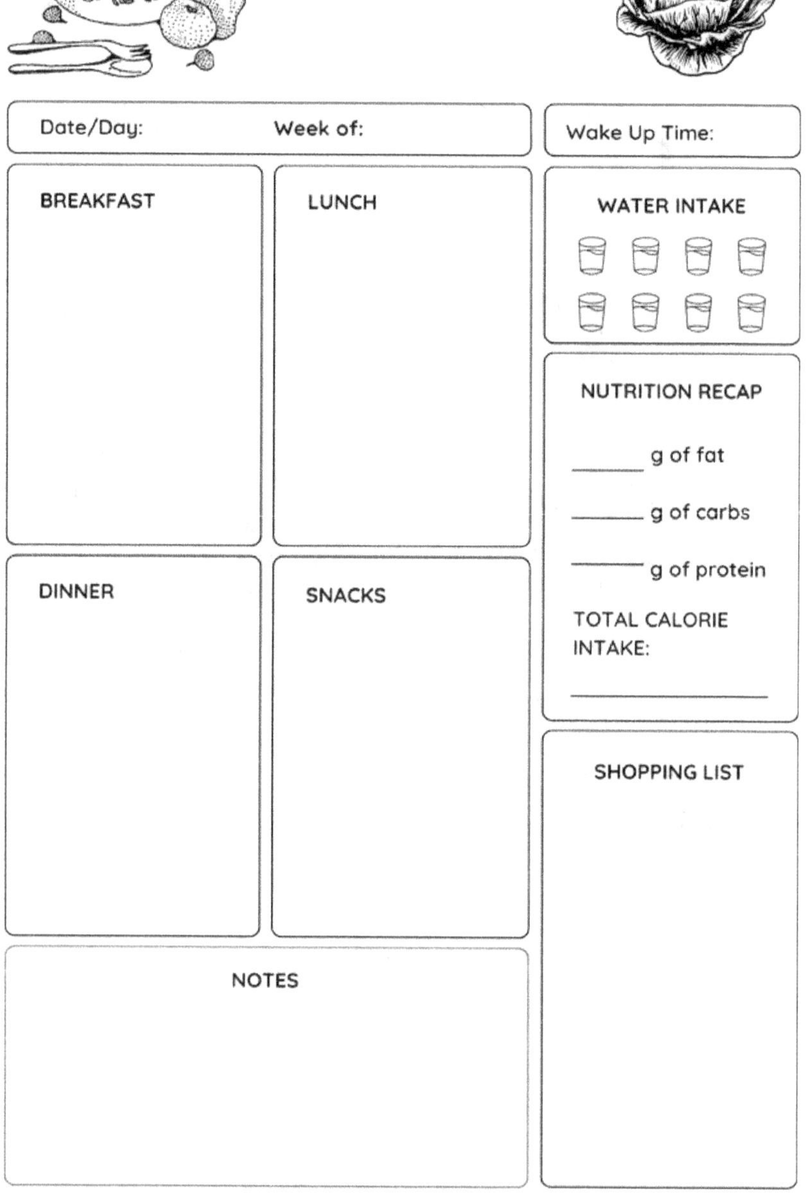

Date/Day:
Week of:
Wake Up Time:
BREAKFAST
LUNCH
WATER INTAKE
NUTRITION RECAP
_______ g of fat
_______ g of carbs
_______ g of protein
TOTAL CALORIE INTAKE:
DINNER
SNACKS
SHOPPING LIST
NOTES

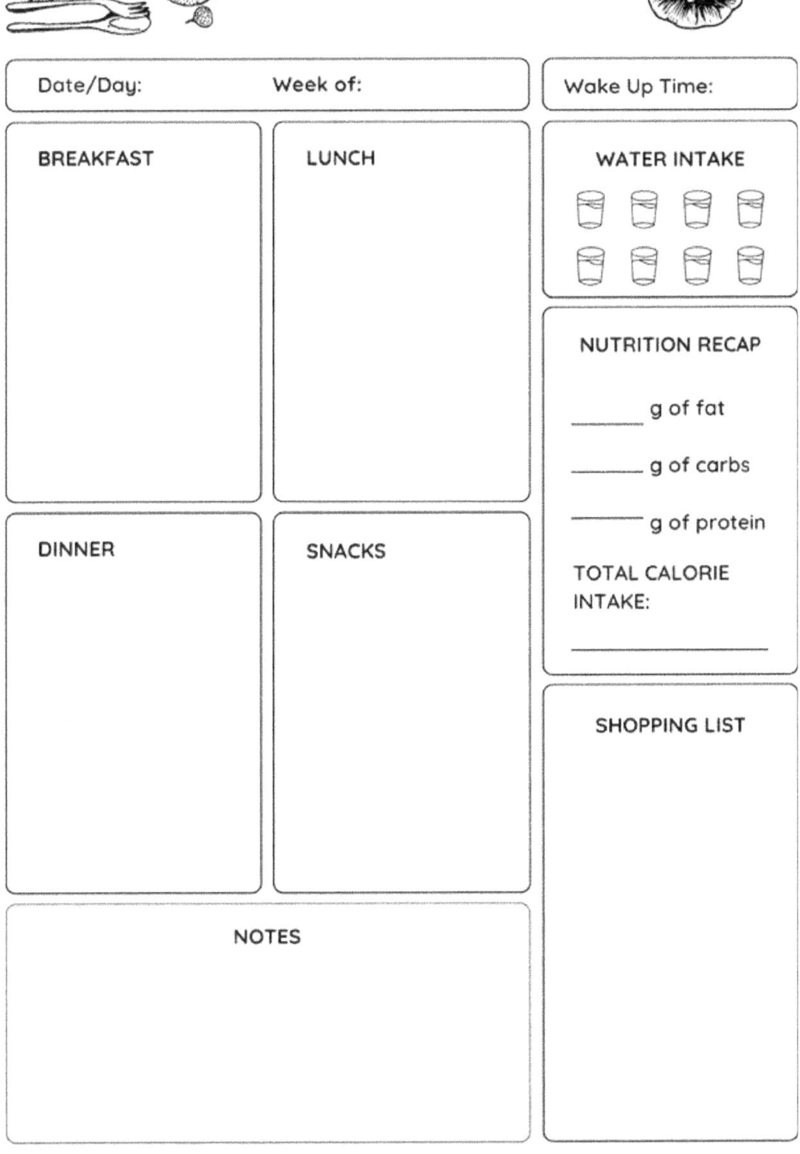

Date/Day:
Week of:
Wake Up Time:

BREAKFAST

LUNCH

WATER INTAKE

NUTRITION RECAP

_______ g of fat

_______ g of carbs

_______ g of protein

TOTAL CALORIE
INTAKE:

DINNER

SNACKS

SHOPPING LIST

NOTES

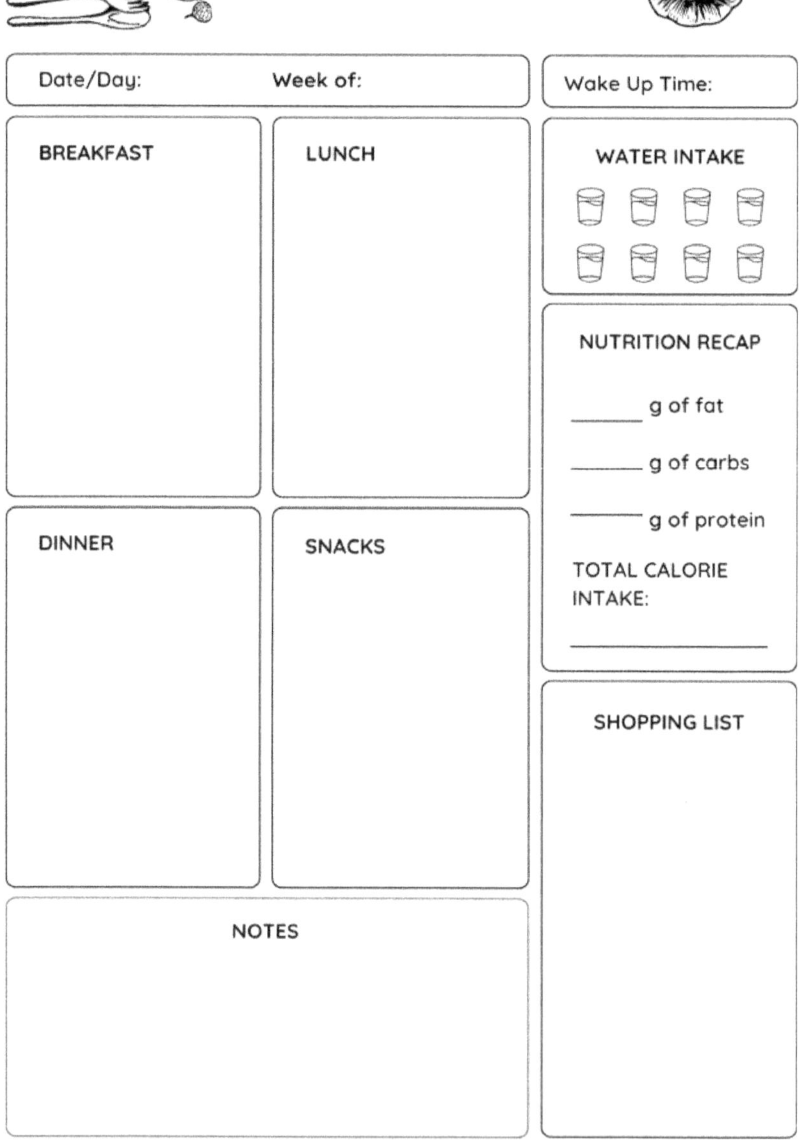

Date/Day: Week of:
Wake Up Time:
BREAKFAST
LUNCH
WATER INTAKE
NUTRITION RECAP
______ g of fat
______ g of carbs
______ g of protein
TOTAL CALORIE INTAKE:
DINNER
SNACKS
SHOPPING LIST
NOTES

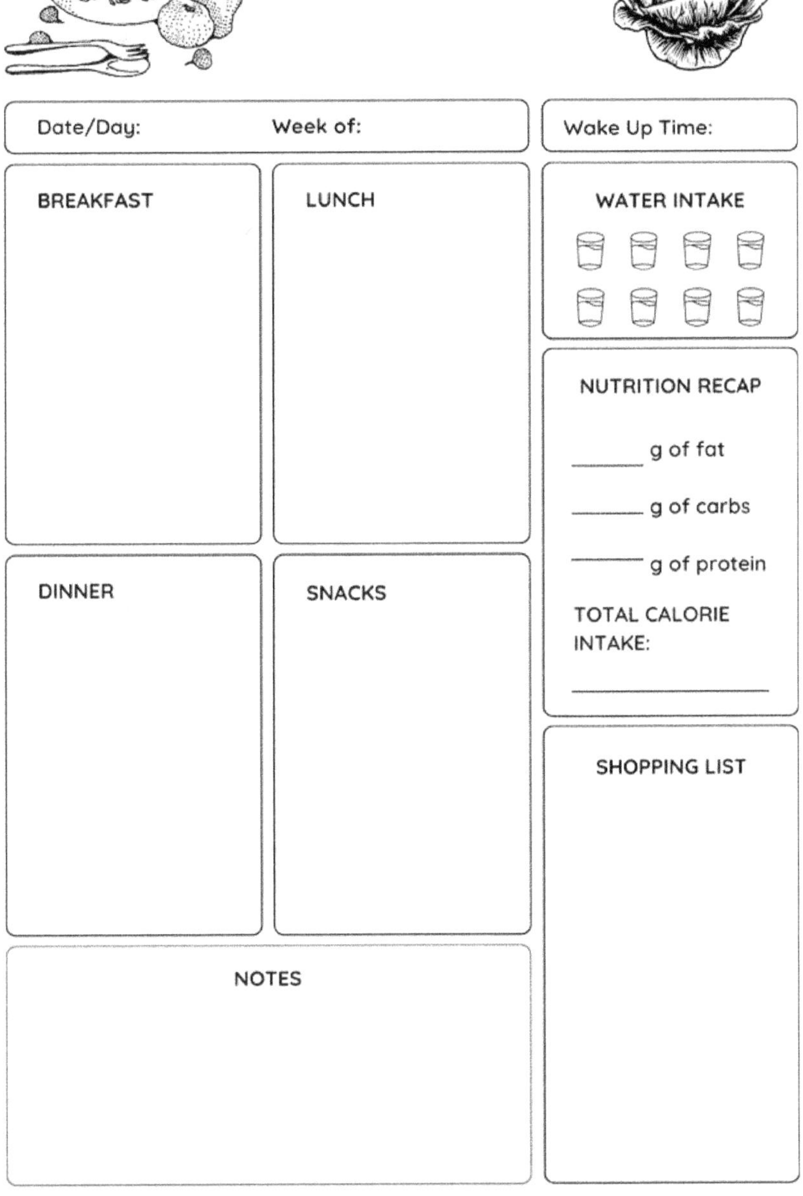

| Date/Day: | Week of: | Wake Up Time: |

BREAKFAST

LUNCH

WATER INTAKE

NUTRITION RECAP

_______ g of fat

_______ g of carbs

_______ g of protein

TOTAL CALORIE INTAKE:

____

DINNER

SNACKS

SHOPPING LIST

NOTES

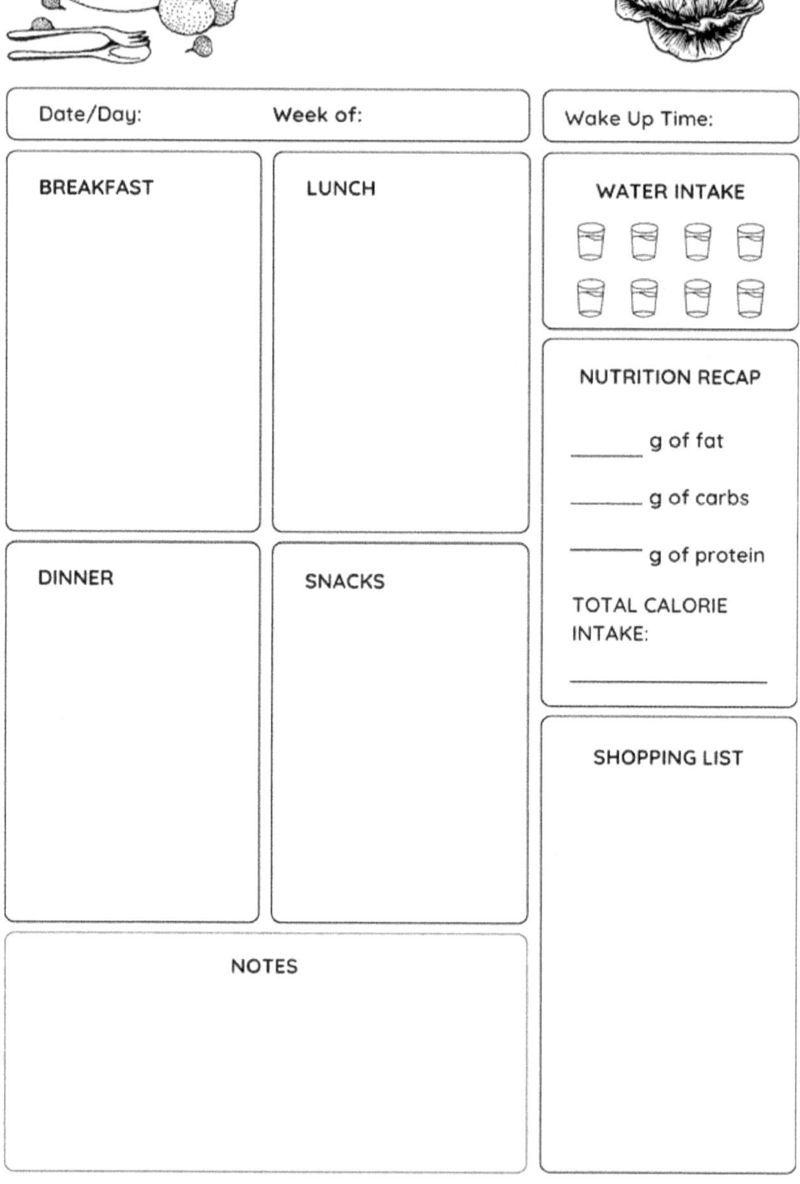

Date/Day: Week of:

Wake Up Time:

BREAKFAST

LUNCH

WATER INTAKE

NUTRITION RECAP

_______ g of fat

_______ g of carbs

_______ g of protein

TOTAL CALORIE INTAKE:

____

DINNER

SNACKS

SHOPPING LIST

NOTES

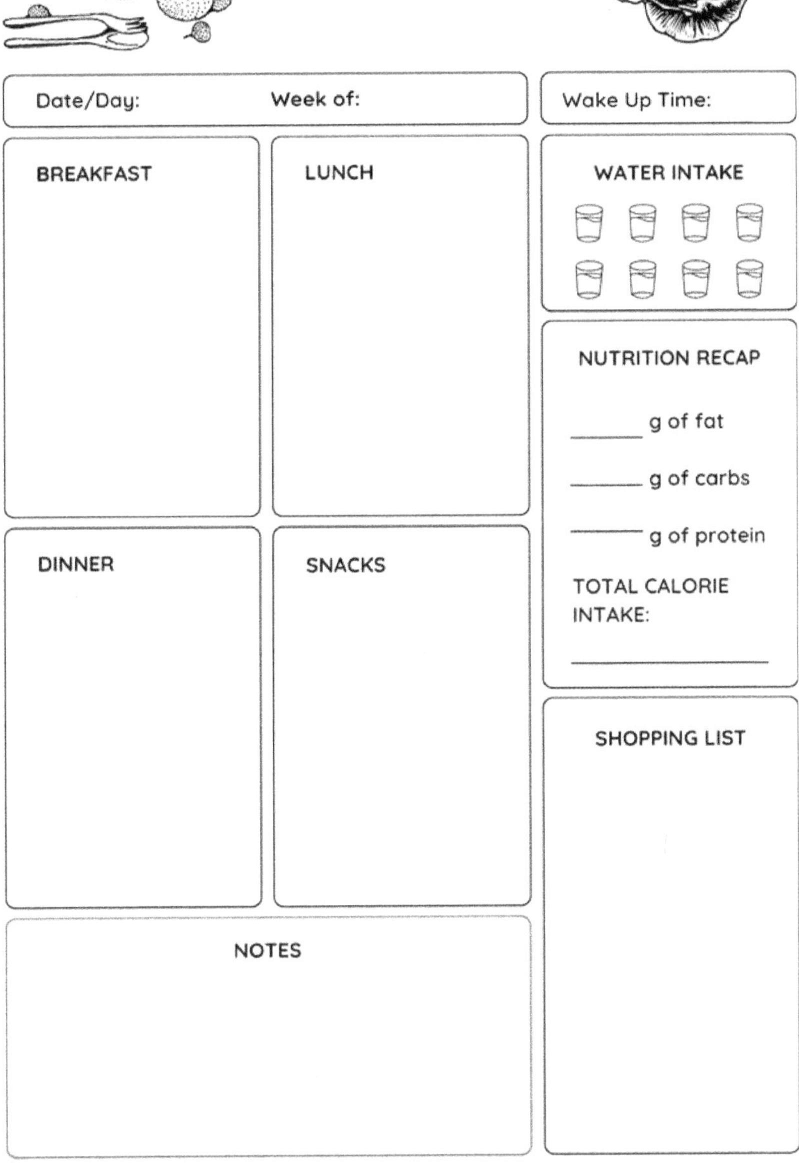

| Date/Day: | Week of: | Wake Up Time: |

BREAKFAST

LUNCH

WATER INTAKE

NUTRITION RECAP

_______ g of fat

_______ g of carbs

_______ g of protein

TOTAL CALORIE INTAKE:

DINNER

SNACKS

SHOPPING LIST

NOTES

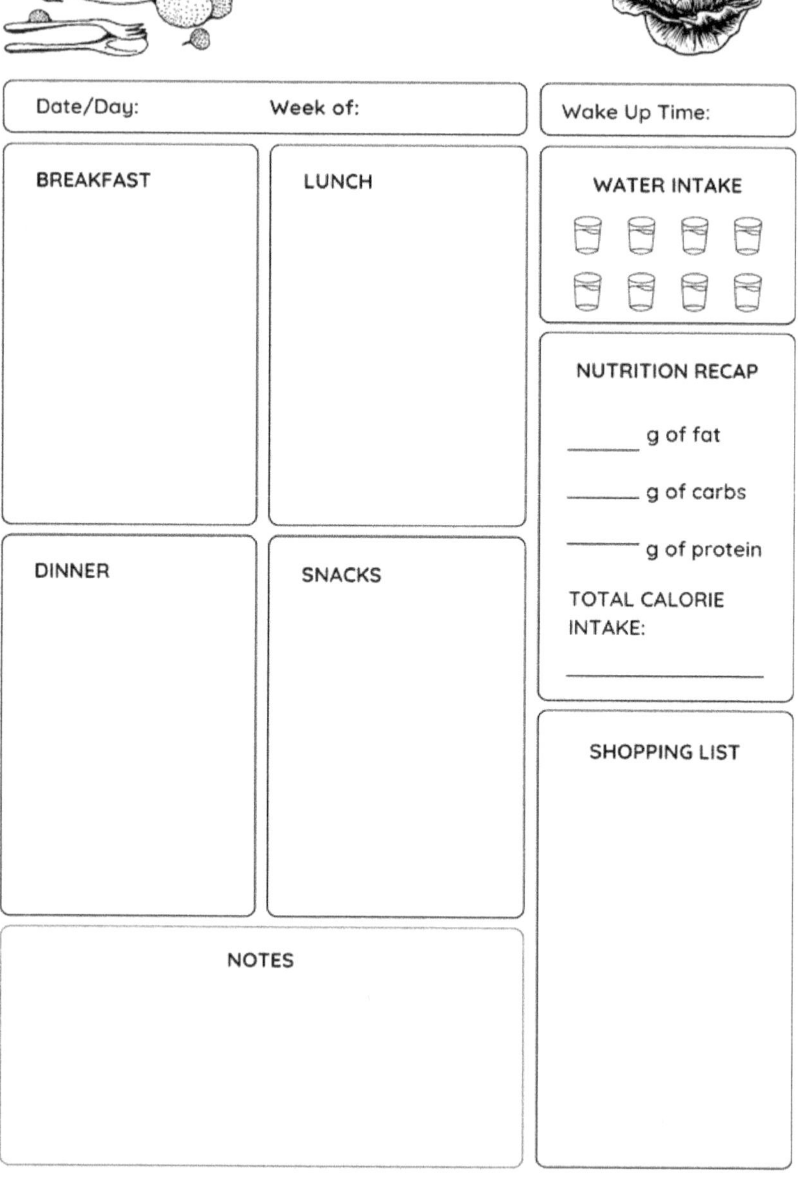

Date/Day:	Week of:

Wake Up Time:

BREAKFAST

LUNCH

WATER INTAKE

DINNER

SNACKS

NUTRITION RECAP

________ g of fat

________ g of carbs

________ g of protein

TOTAL CALORIE INTAKE:

____

SHOPPING LIST

NOTES

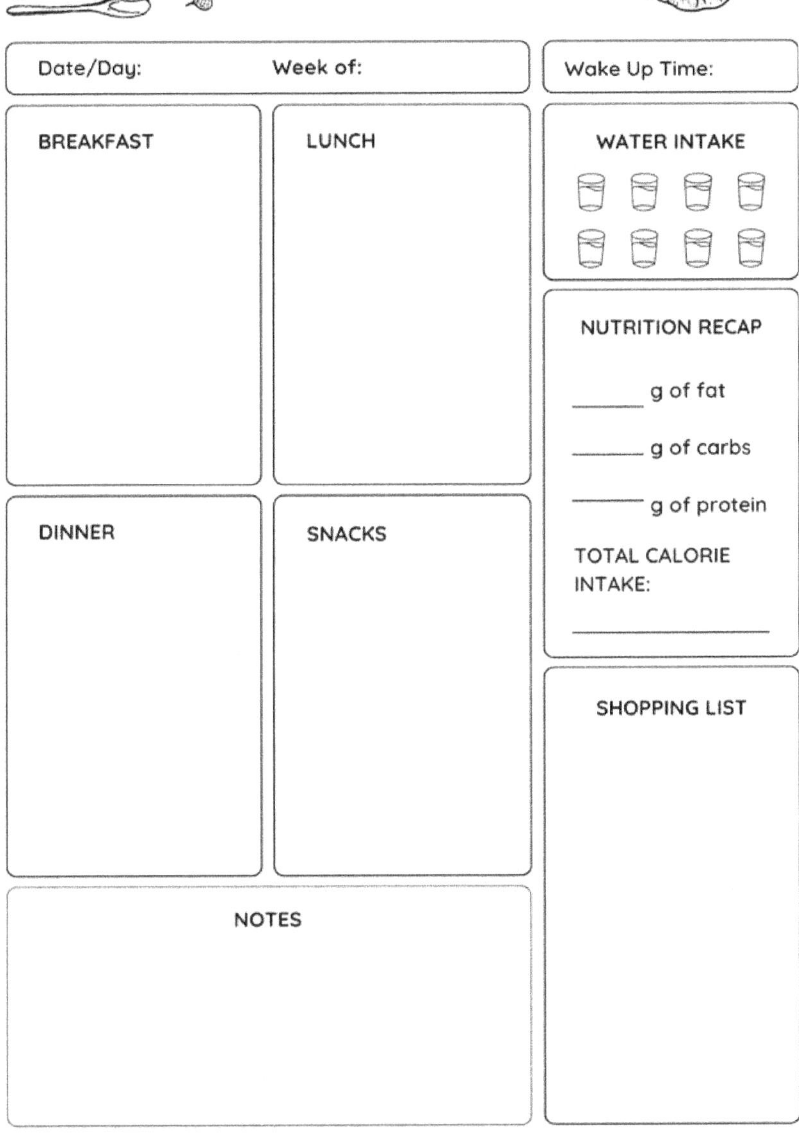

| Date/Day: | Week of: | Wake Up Time: |

BREAKFAST

LUNCH

WATER INTAKE

NUTRITION RECAP

_______ g of fat

_______ g of carbs

_______ g of protein

TOTAL CALORIE INTAKE:

____

DINNER

SNACKS

SHOPPING LIST

NOTES

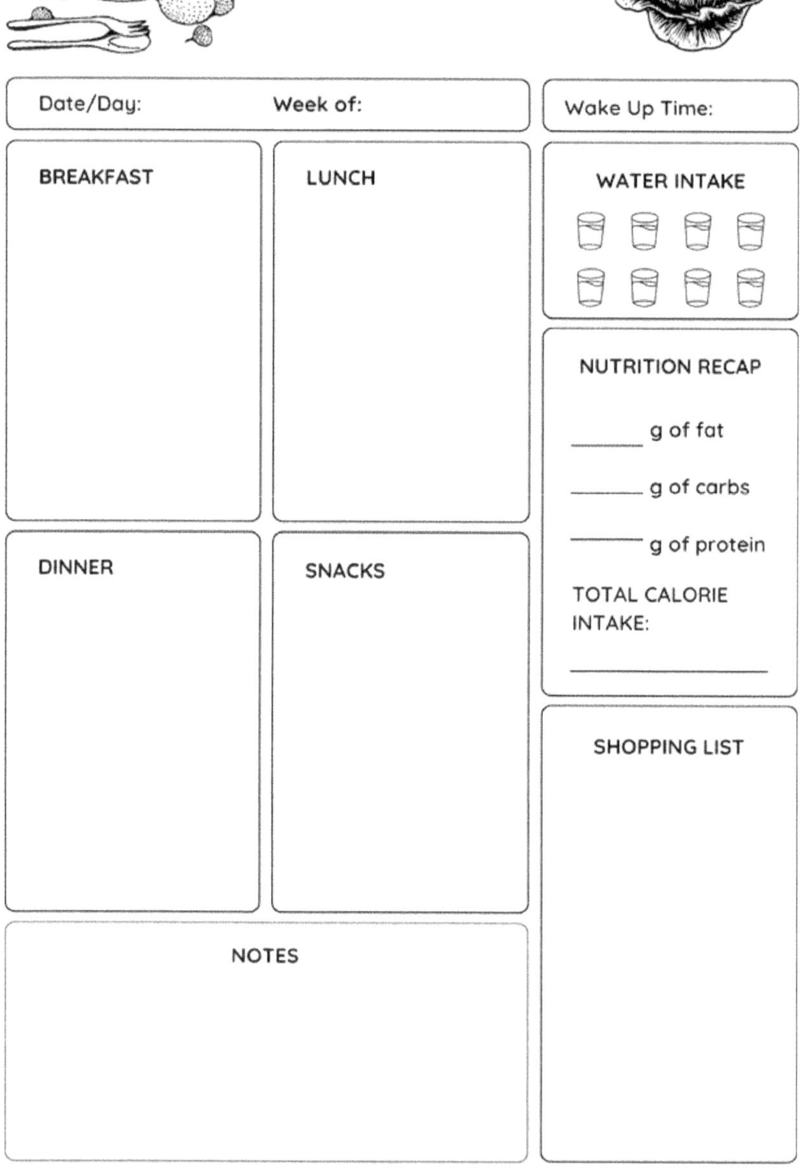

Date/Day: Week of:

Wake Up Time:

BREAKFAST

LUNCH

WATER INTAKE

NUTRITION RECAP

_________ g of fat

_________ g of carbs

_________ g of protein

TOTAL CALORIE INTAKE:

____

DINNER

SNACKS

SHOPPING LIST

NOTES

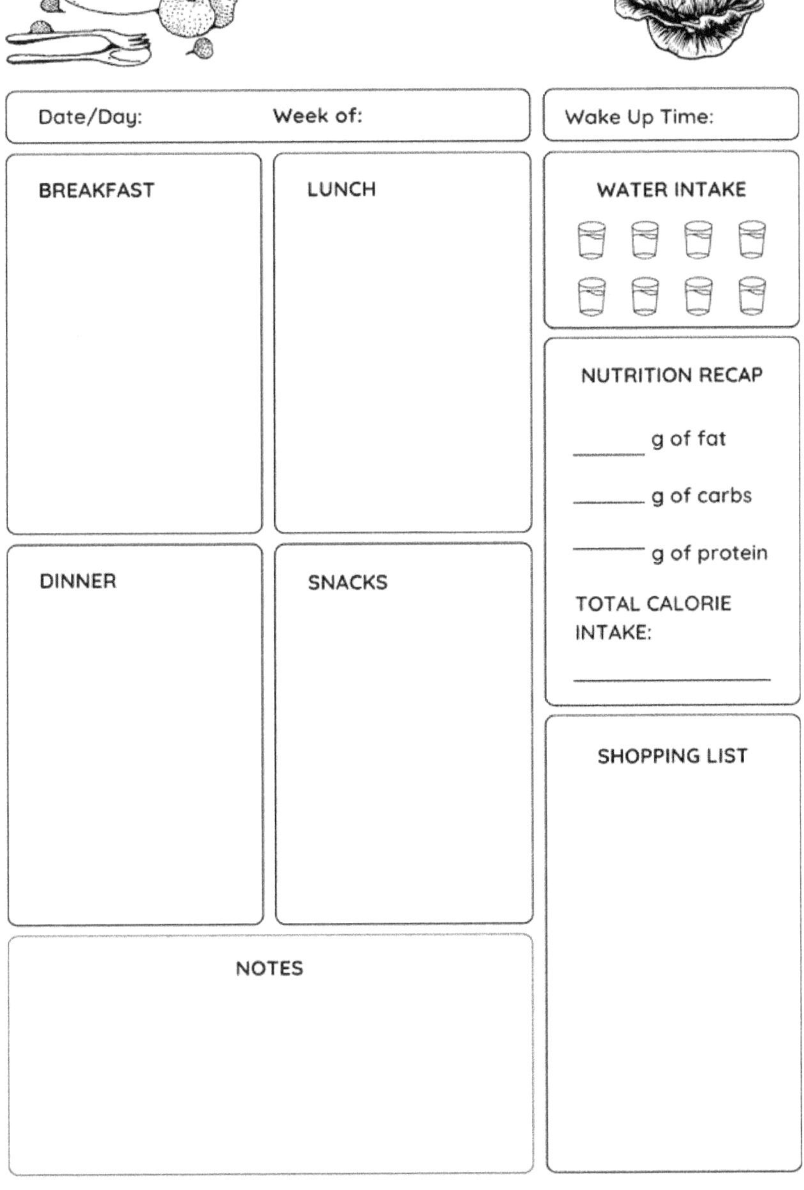

| Date/Day: | Week of: | Wake Up Time: |

BREAKFAST

LUNCH

WATER INTAKE

NUTRITION RECAP

_________ g of fat

_________ g of carbs

_________ g of protein

TOTAL CALORIE INTAKE:

____

DINNER

SNACKS

SHOPPING LIST

NOTES

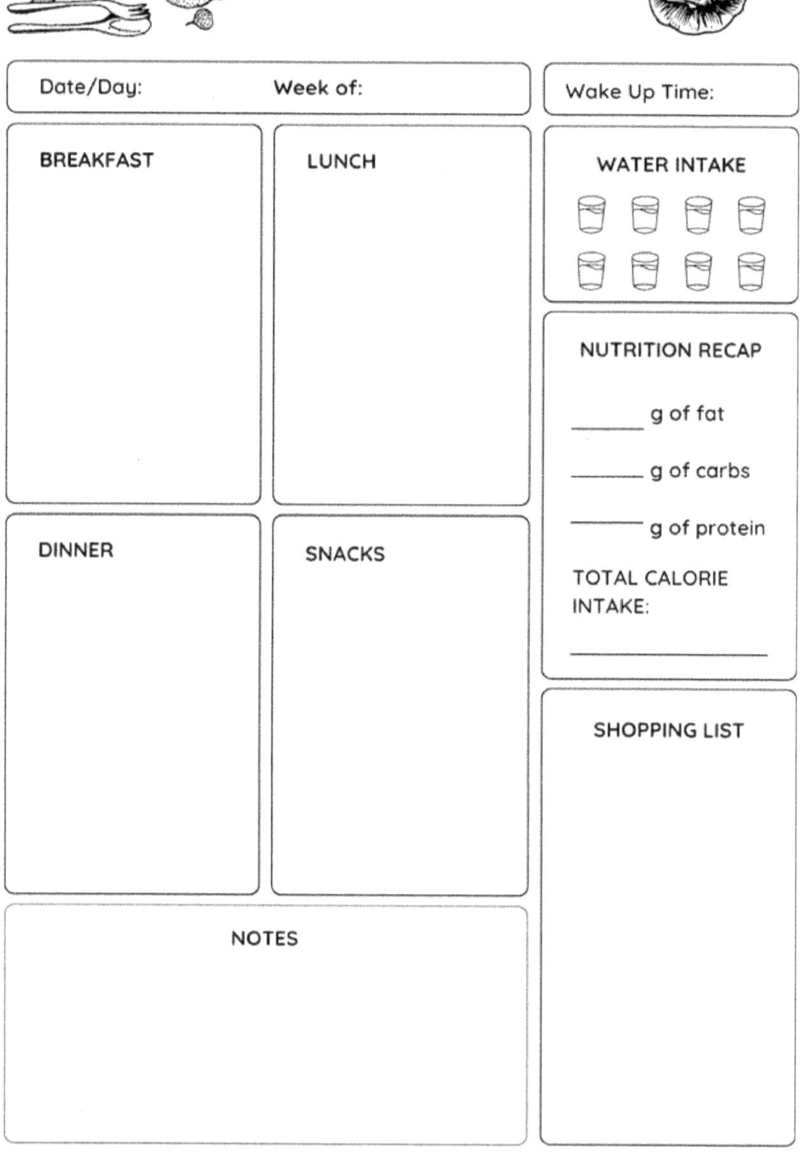

Date/Day:
Week of:
Wake Up Time:
BREAKFAST
LUNCH
WATER INTAKE
NUTRITION RECAP
______ g of fat
______ g of carbs
______ g of protein
TOTAL CALORIE INTAKE:
DINNER
SNACKS
SHOPPING LIST
NOTES

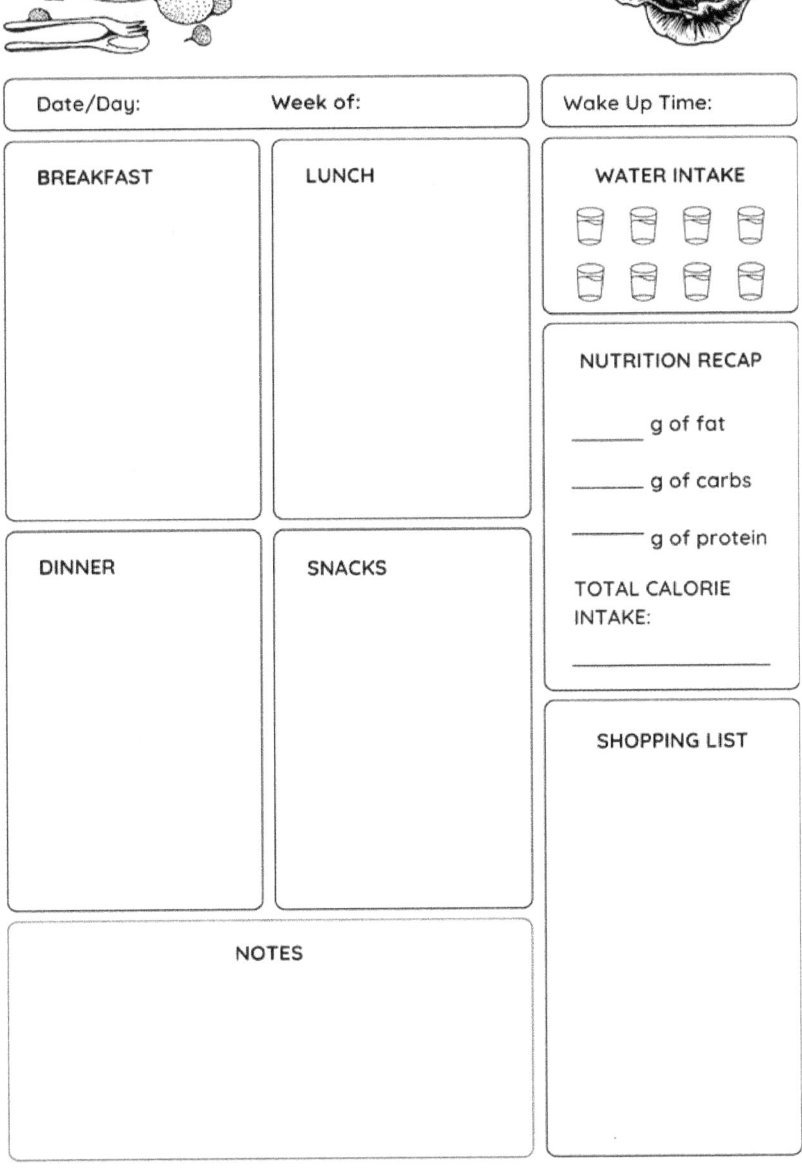

Date/Day: Week of: Wake Up Time:

BREAKFAST

LUNCH

WATER INTAKE

NUTRITION RECAP

______ g of fat

______ g of carbs

______ g of protein

TOTAL CALORIE INTAKE:

DINNER

SNACKS

SHOPPING LIST

NOTES

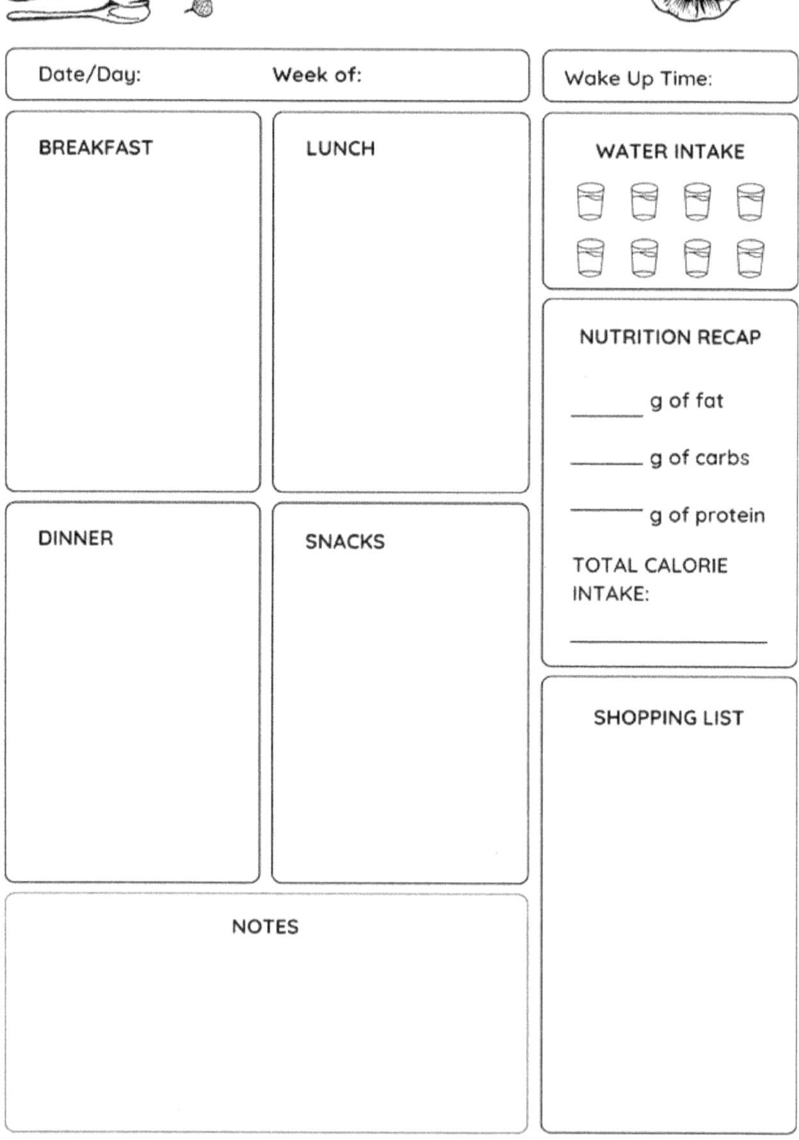

| Date/Day: | Week of: | Wake Up Time: |

BREAKFAST

LUNCH

WATER INTAKE

NUTRITION RECAP

_______ g of fat

_______ g of carbs

_______ g of protein

TOTAL CALORIE INTAKE:

DINNER

SNACKS

SHOPPING LIST

NOTES

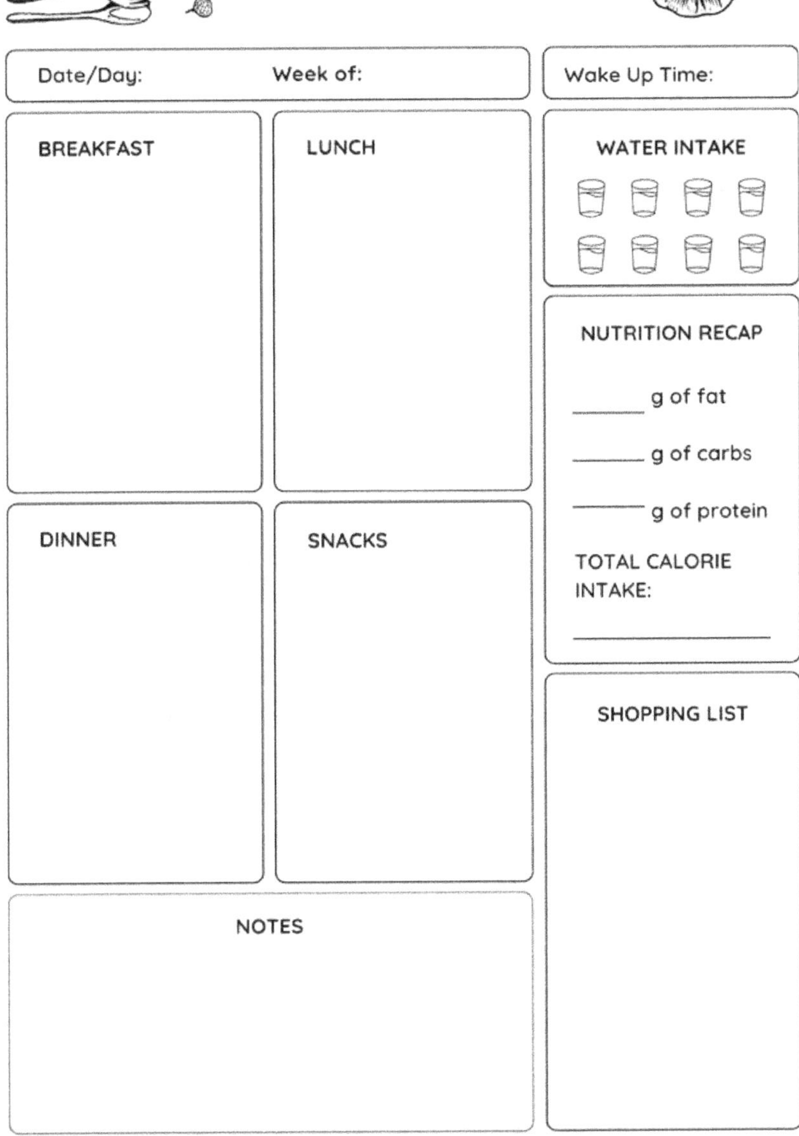

| Date/Day: | Week of: | Wake Up Time: |

BREAKFAST

LUNCH

WATER INTAKE

NUTRITION RECAP

_______ g of fat

_______ g of carbs

_______ g of protein

TOTAL CALORIE INTAKE:

____

DINNER

SNACKS

SHOPPING LIST

NOTES

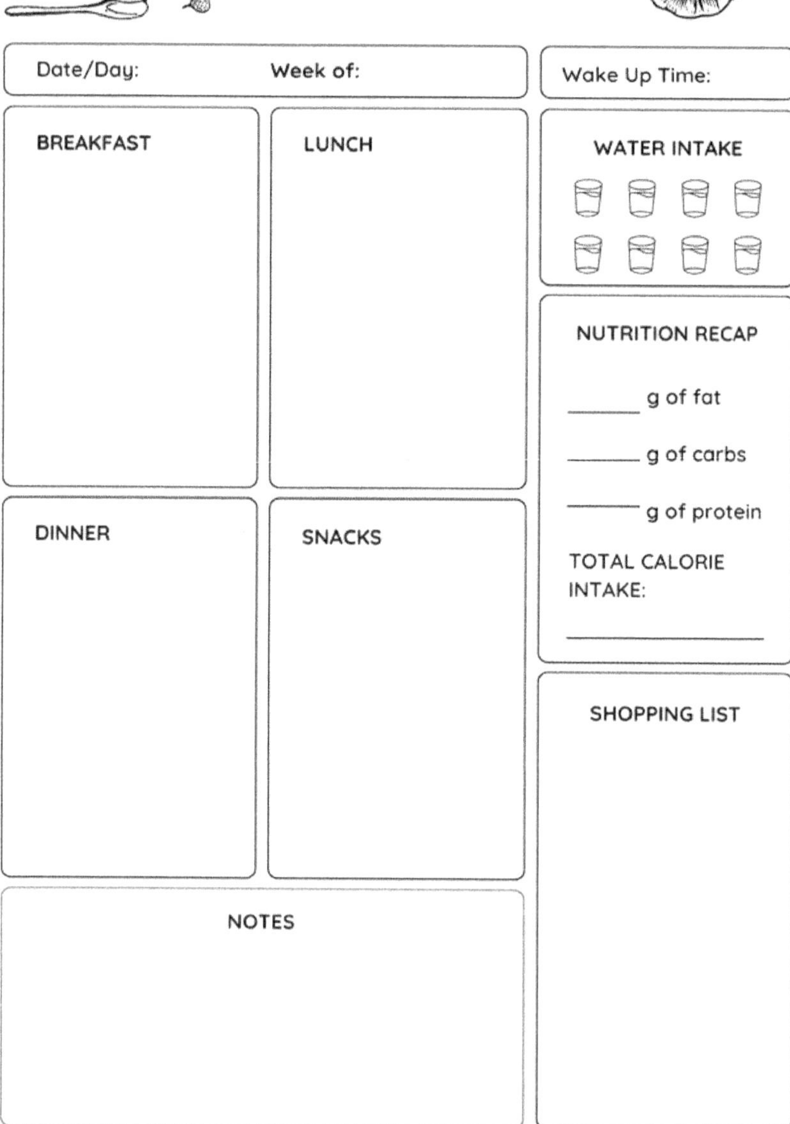

Date/Day:
Week of:
Wake Up Time:
BREAKFAST
LUNCH
WATER INTAKE
NUTRITION RECAP
_______ g of fat
_______ g of carbs
_______ g of protein
TOTAL CALORIE INTAKE:
DINNER
SNACKS
SHOPPING LIST
NOTES

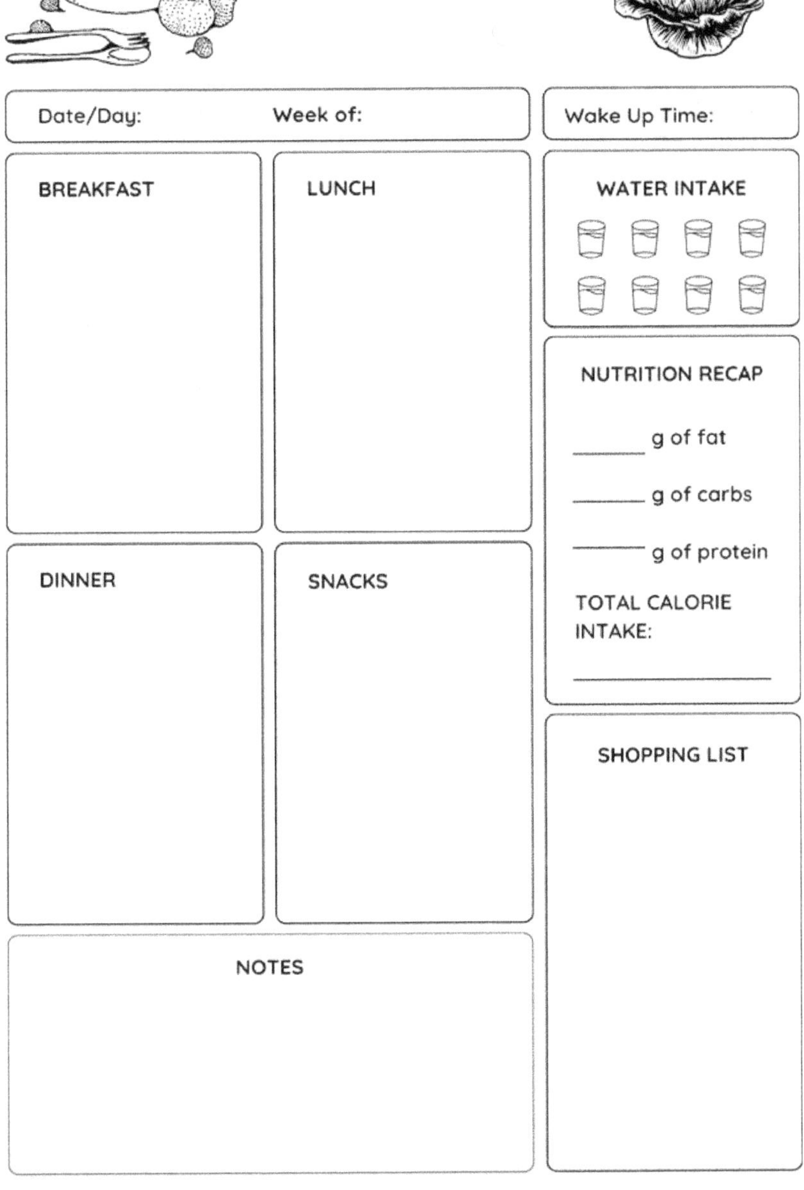

| Date/Day: | Week of: | Wake Up Time: |

BREAKFAST

LUNCH

WATER INTAKE

NUTRITION RECAP

_____ g of fat

_____ g of carbs

_____ g of protein

TOTAL CALORIE INTAKE:

_____

DINNER

SNACKS

SHOPPING LIST

NOTES

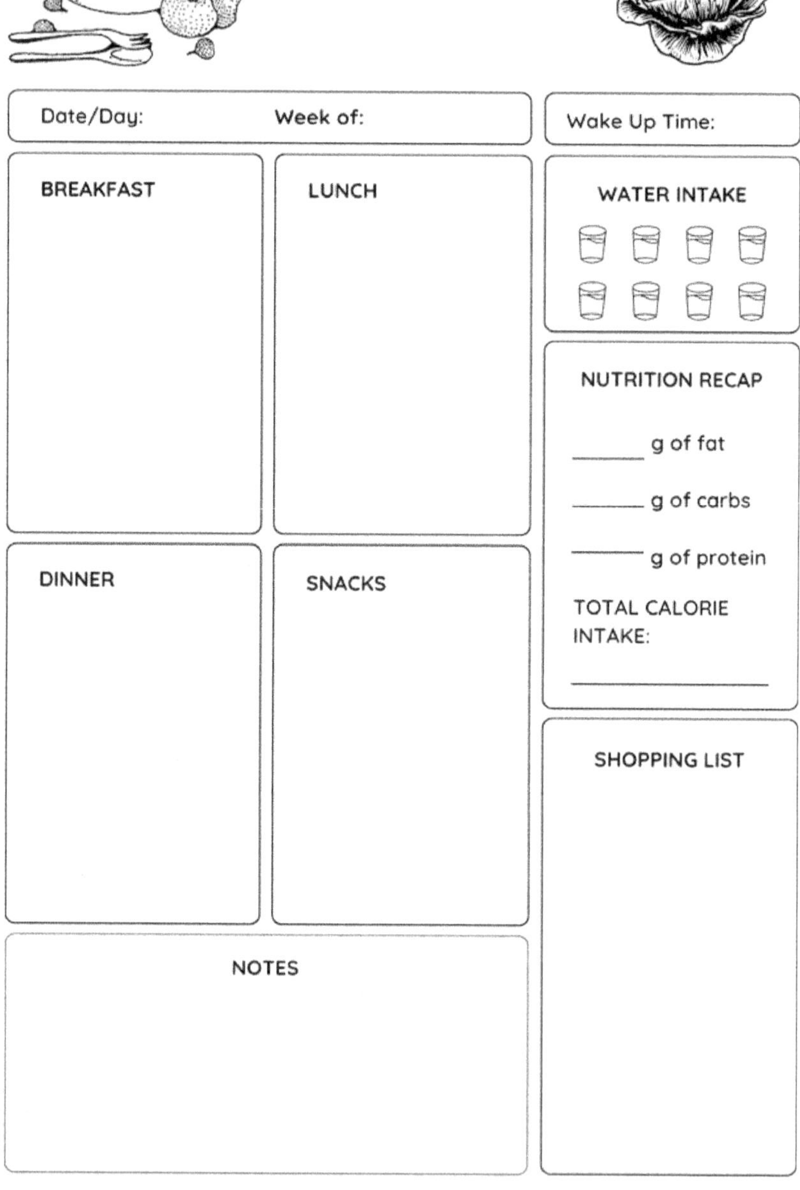

| Date/Day: | Week of: | Wake Up Time: |

BREAKFAST

LUNCH

WATER INTAKE

NUTRITION RECAP

________ g of fat

________ g of carbs

________ g of protein

TOTAL CALORIE INTAKE:

____

DINNER

SNACKS

SHOPPING LIST

NOTES

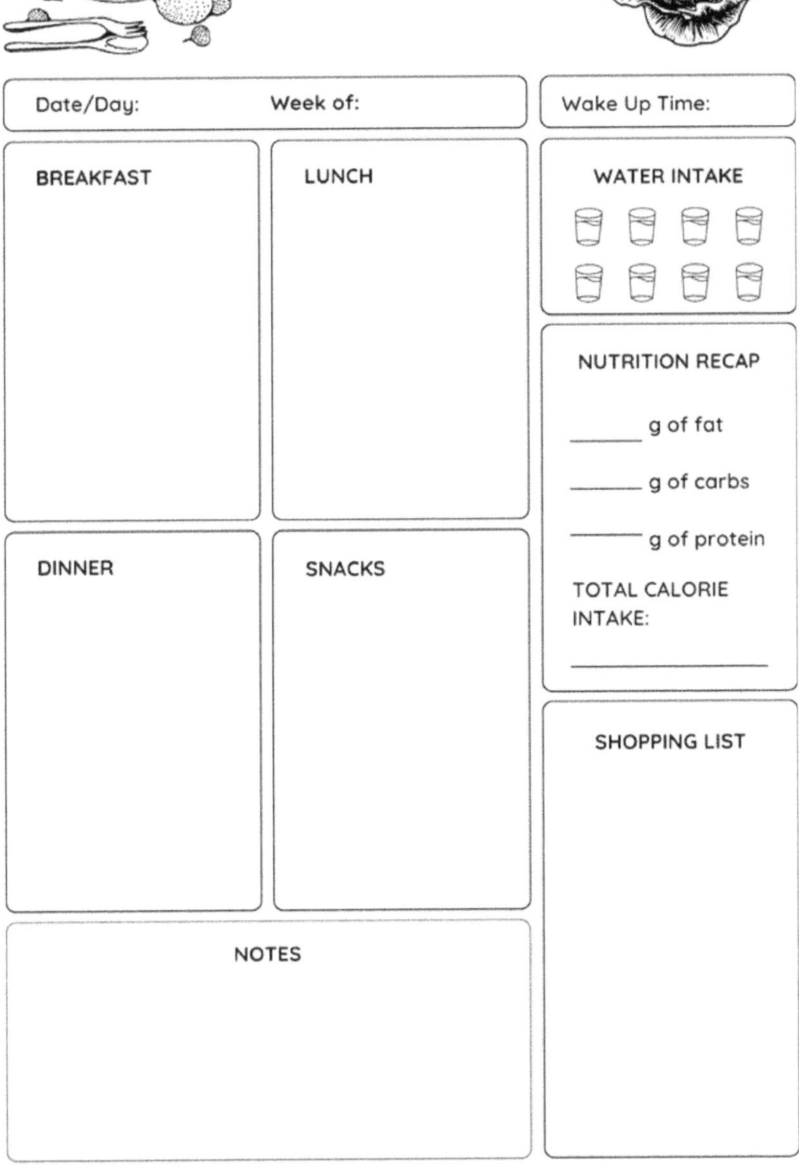
Date/Day:
Week of:
Wake Up Time:
BREAKFAST
LUNCH
WATER INTAKE
NUTRITION RECAP
_______ g of fat
_______ g of carbs
_______ g of protein
TOTAL CALORIE INTAKE:
DINNER
SNACKS
SHOPPING LIST
NOTES

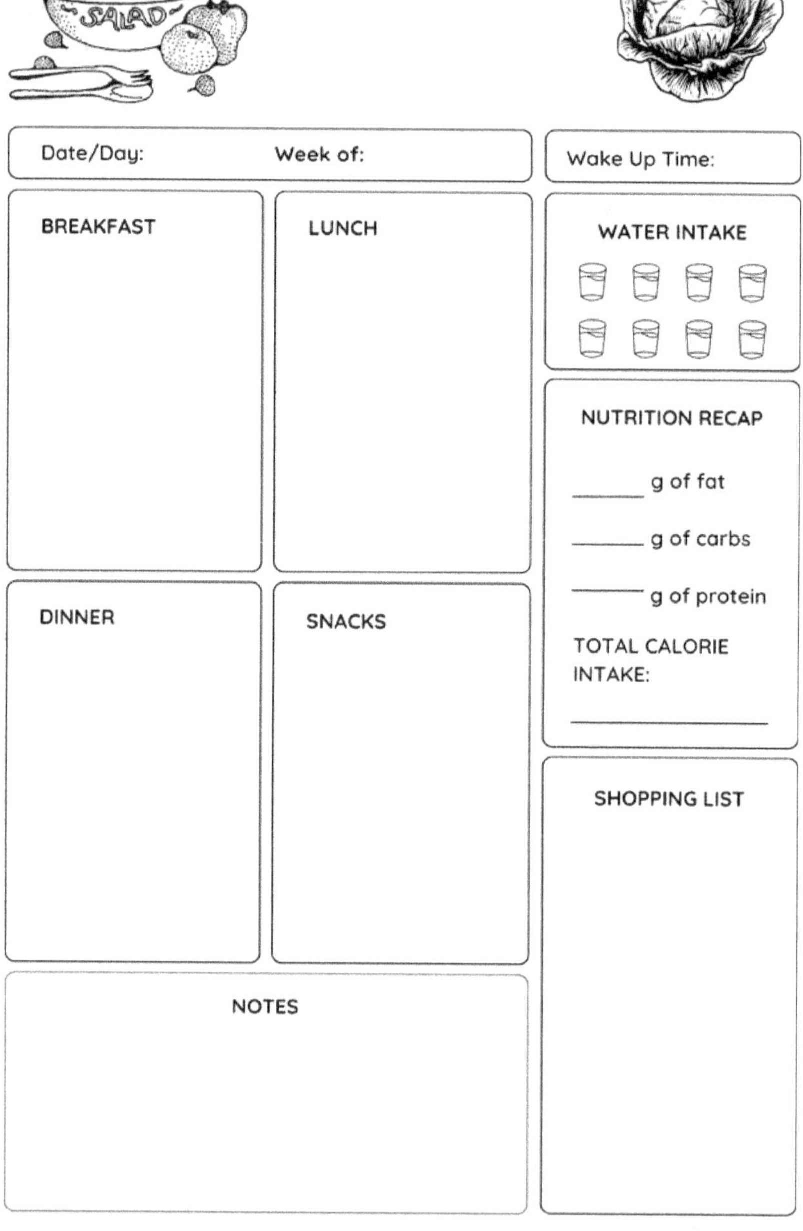
Date/Day:
Week of:
Wake Up Time:
BREAKFAST
LUNCH
WATER INTAKE
NUTRITION RECAP
_______ g of fat
_______ g of carbs
_______ g of protein
TOTAL CALORIE INTAKE:
DINNER
SNACKS
SHOPPING LIST
NOTES

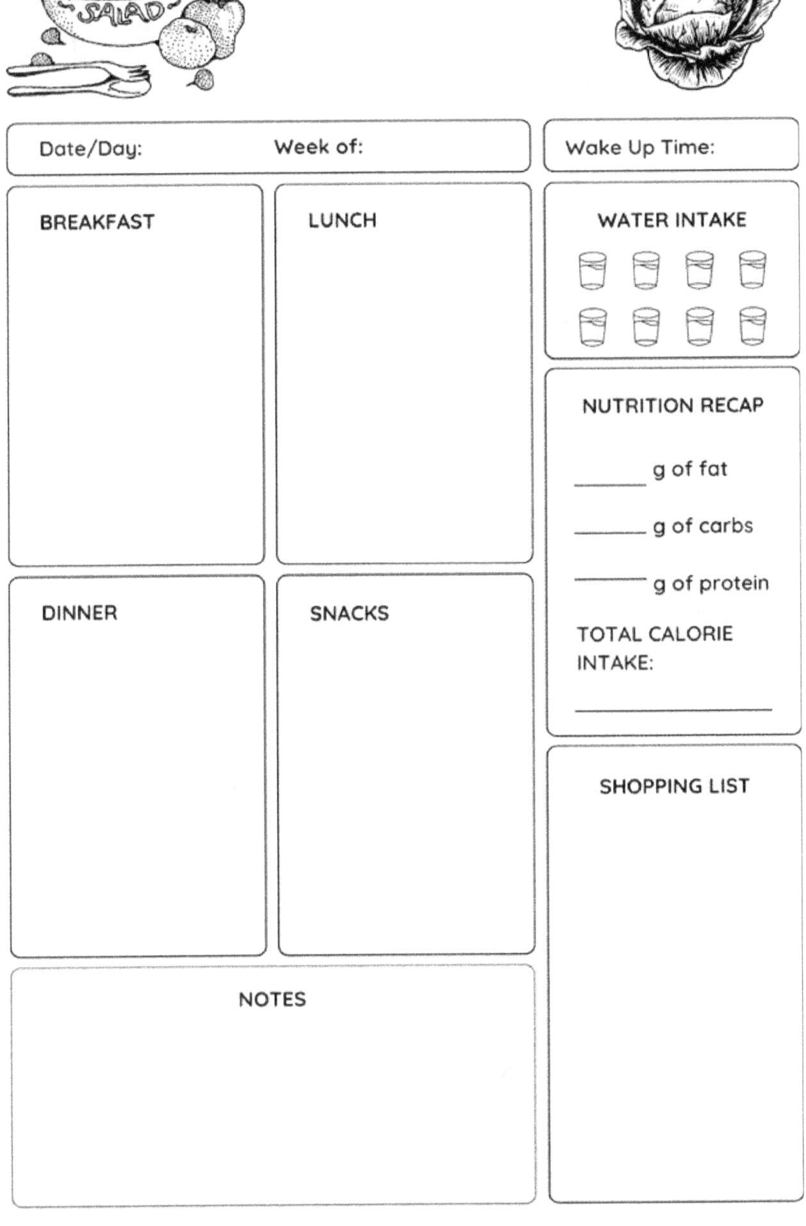

Date/Day:
Week of:
Wake Up Time:
BREAKFAST
LUNCH
WATER INTAKE
NUTRITION RECAP
_______ g of fat
_______ g of carbs
_______ g of protein
TOTAL CALORIE INTAKE:
DINNER
SNACKS
SHOPPING LIST
NOTES

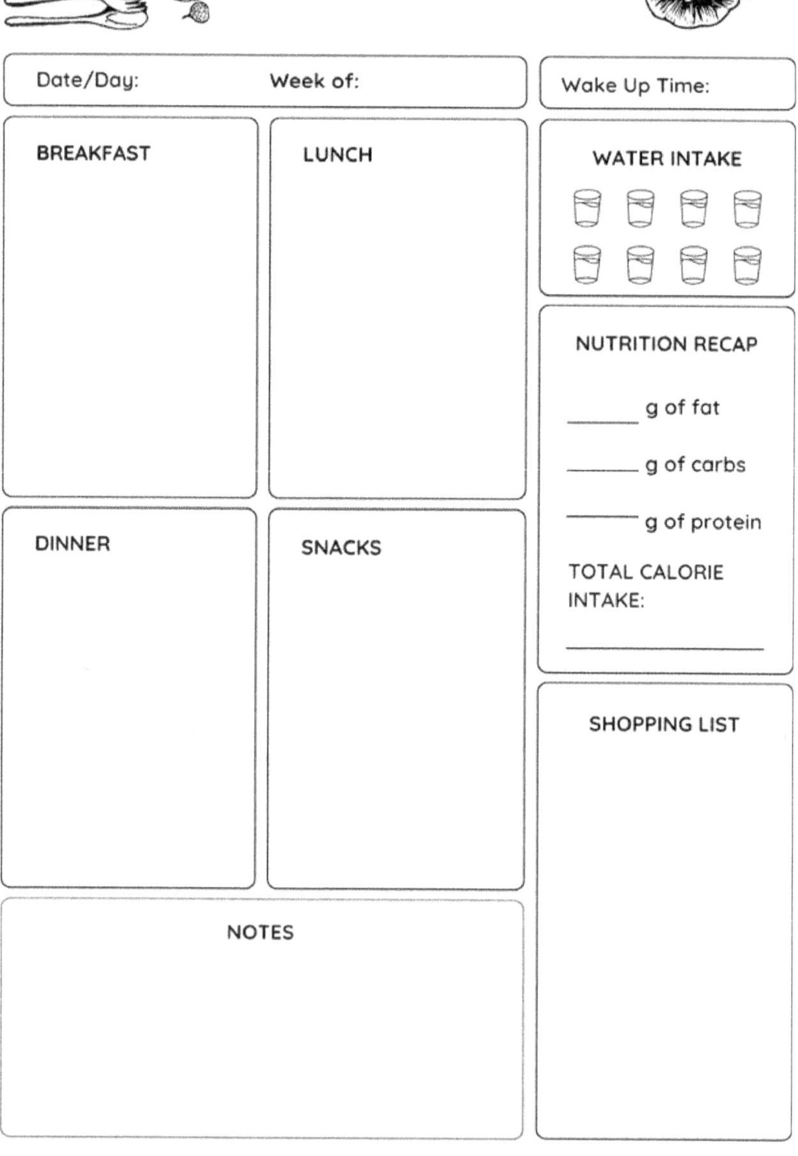

Date/Day: Week of:
Wake Up Time:
BREAKFAST
LUNCH
WATER INTAKE
NUTRITION RECAP
_______ g of fat
_______ g of carbs
_______ g of protein
TOTAL CALORIE
INTAKE:
____
DINNER
SNACKS
SHOPPING LIST
NOTES

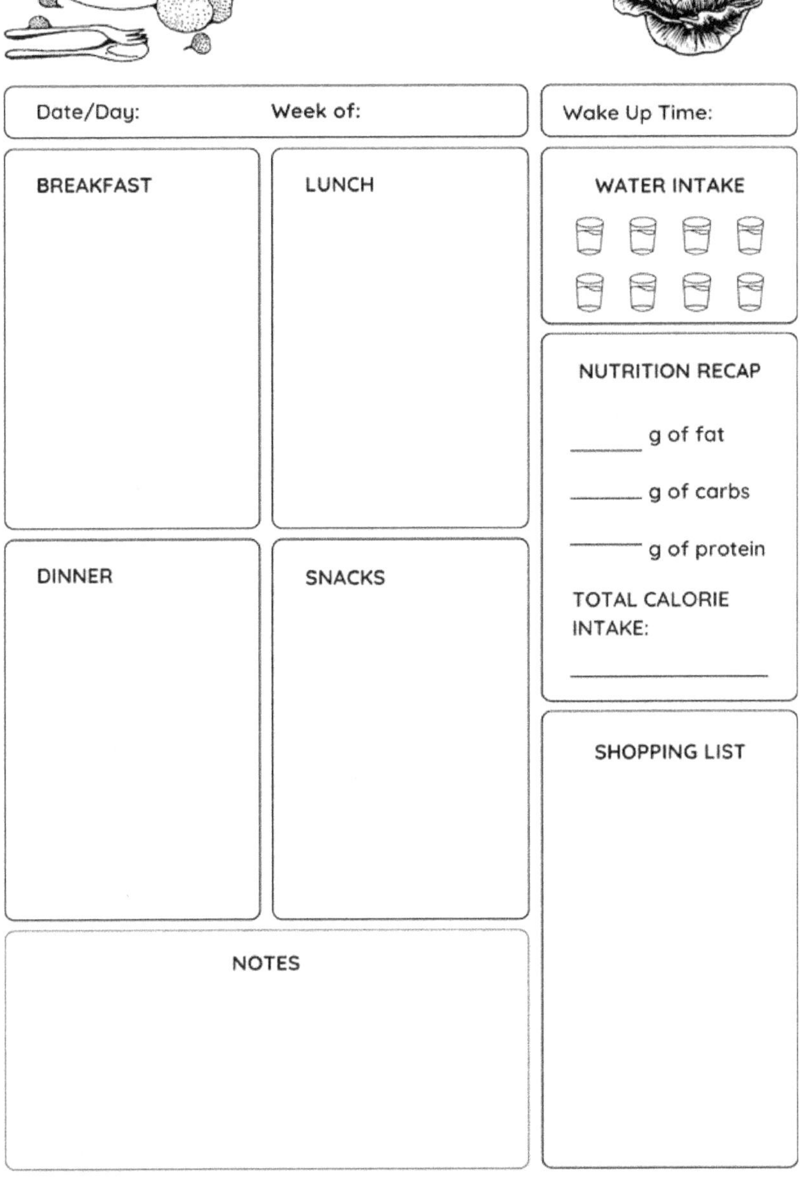

Date/Day:	Week of:

Wake Up Time:

BREAKFAST

LUNCH

WATER INTAKE

NUTRITION RECAP

_________ g of fat

_________ g of carbs

_________ g of protein

TOTAL CALORIE INTAKE:

____

DINNER

SNACKS

SHOPPING LIST

NOTES

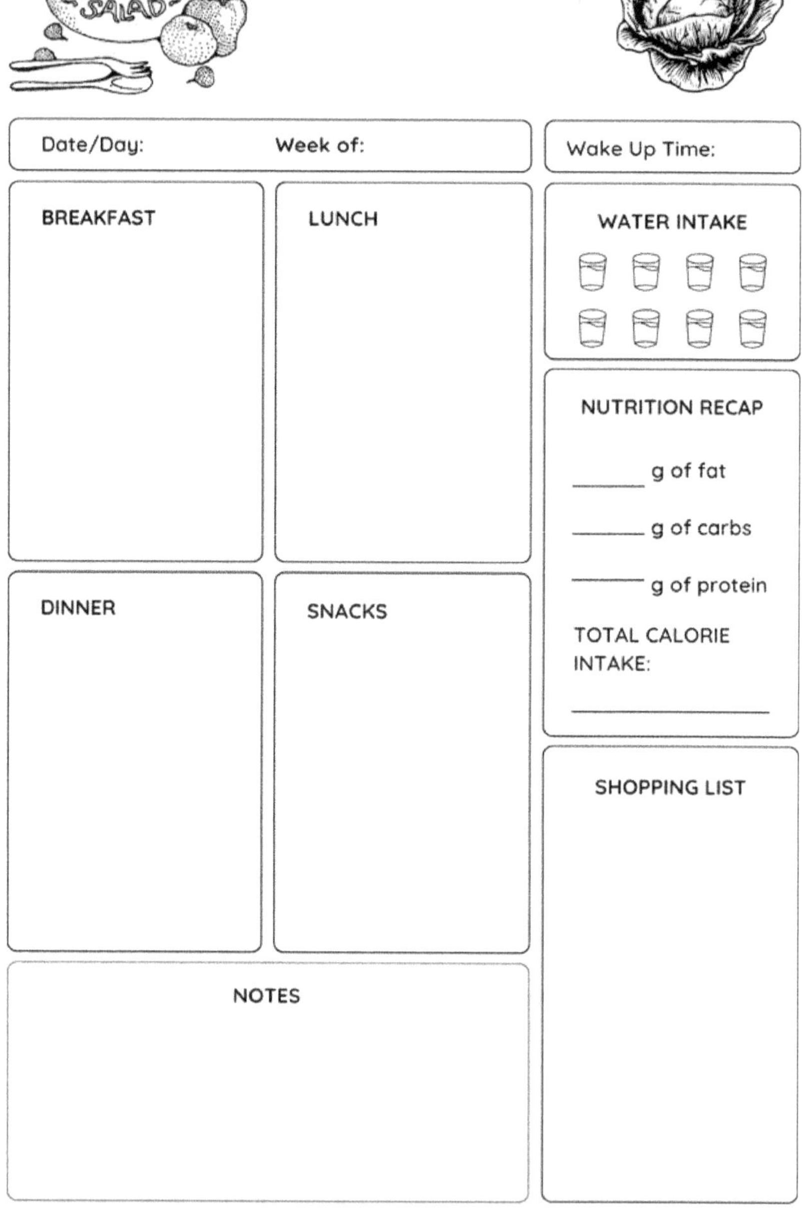

Date/Day: **Week of:**

Wake Up Time:

BREAKFAST

LUNCH

WATER INTAKE

NUTRITION RECAP

________ g of fat

________ g of carbs

________ g of protein

TOTAL CALORIE INTAKE:

____

DINNER

SNACKS

SHOPPING LIST

NOTES

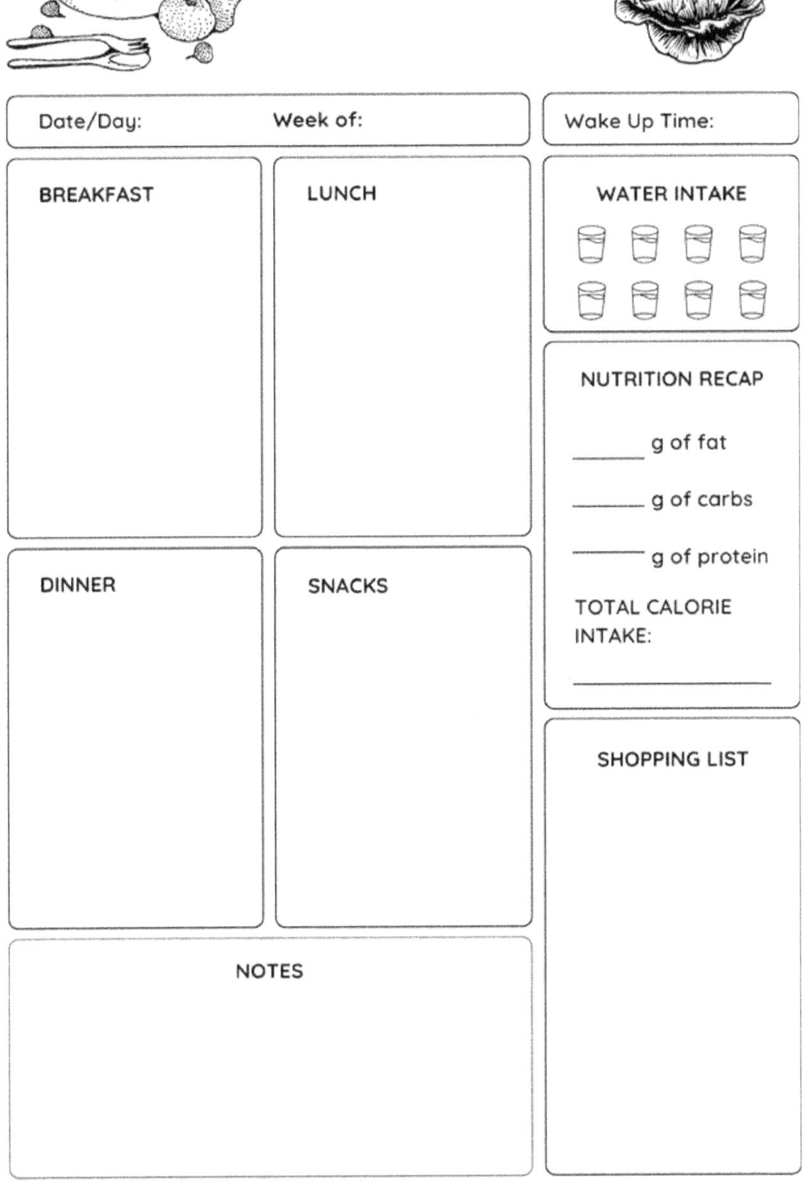

Date/Day: Week of:
Wake Up Time:
BREAKFAST
LUNCH
WATER INTAKE
NUTRITION RECAP
______ g of fat
______ g of carbs
______ g of protein
TOTAL CALORIE INTAKE:
DINNER
SNACKS
SHOPPING LIST
NOTES

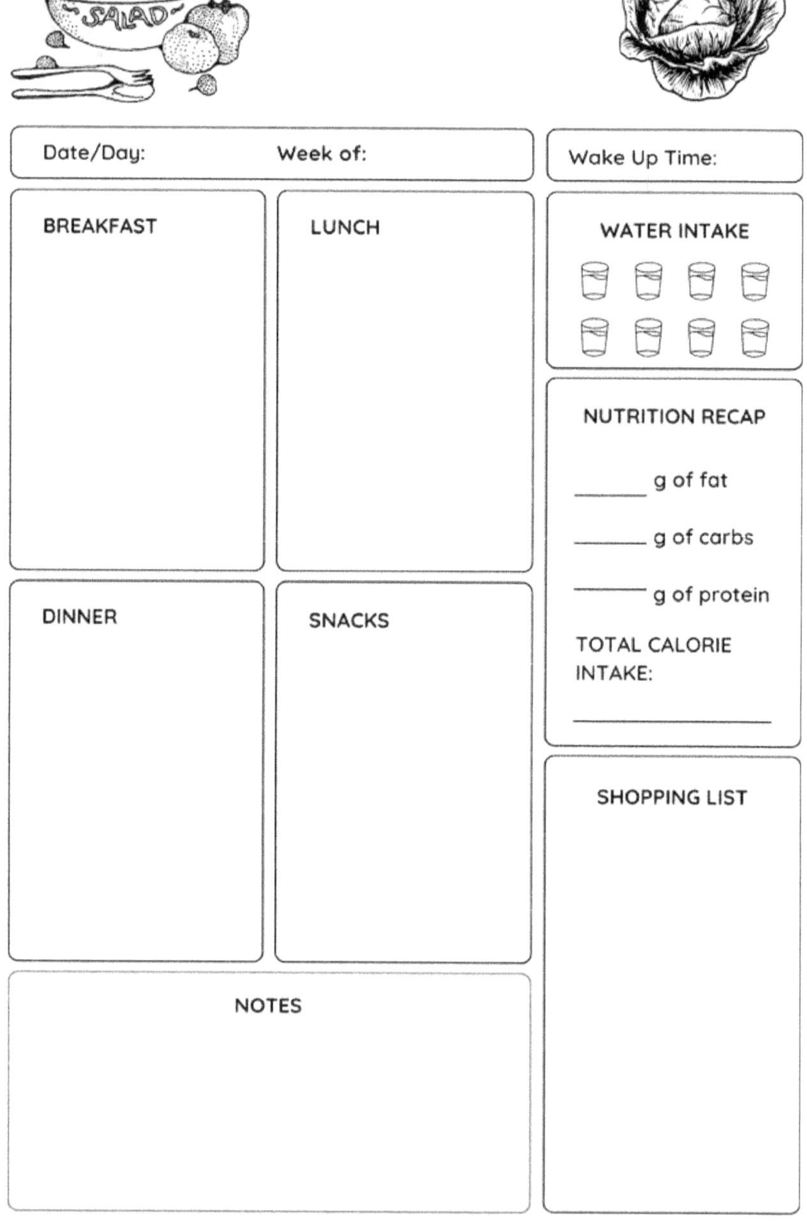

Date/Day:
Week of:
Wake Up Time:
BREAKFAST
LUNCH
WATER INTAKE
NUTRITION RECAP
_______ g of fat
_______ g of carbs
_______ g of protein
TOTAL CALORIE INTAKE:
DINNER
SNACKS
SHOPPING LIST
NOTES

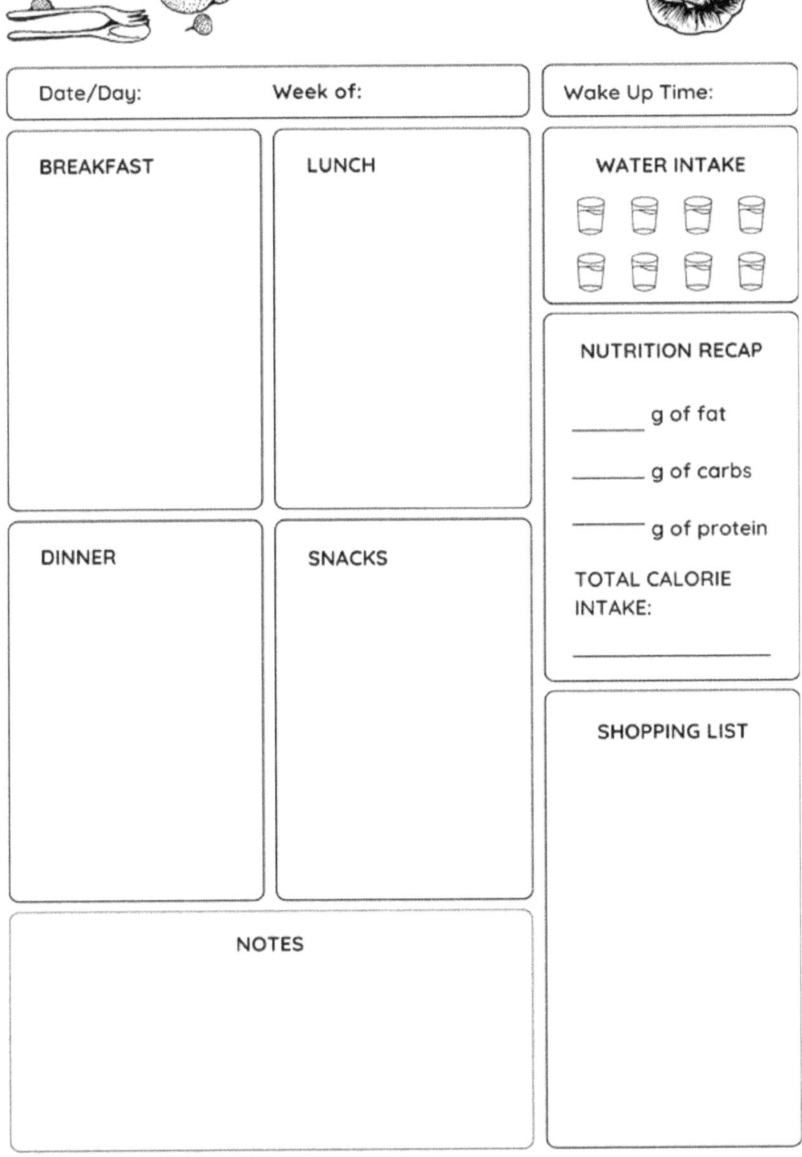

| Date/Day: | Week of: | Wake Up Time: |

BREAKFAST

LUNCH

WATER INTAKE

NUTRITION RECAP

________ g of fat

________ g of carbs

________ g of protein

TOTAL CALORIE INTAKE:

DINNER

SNACKS

SHOPPING LIST

NOTES

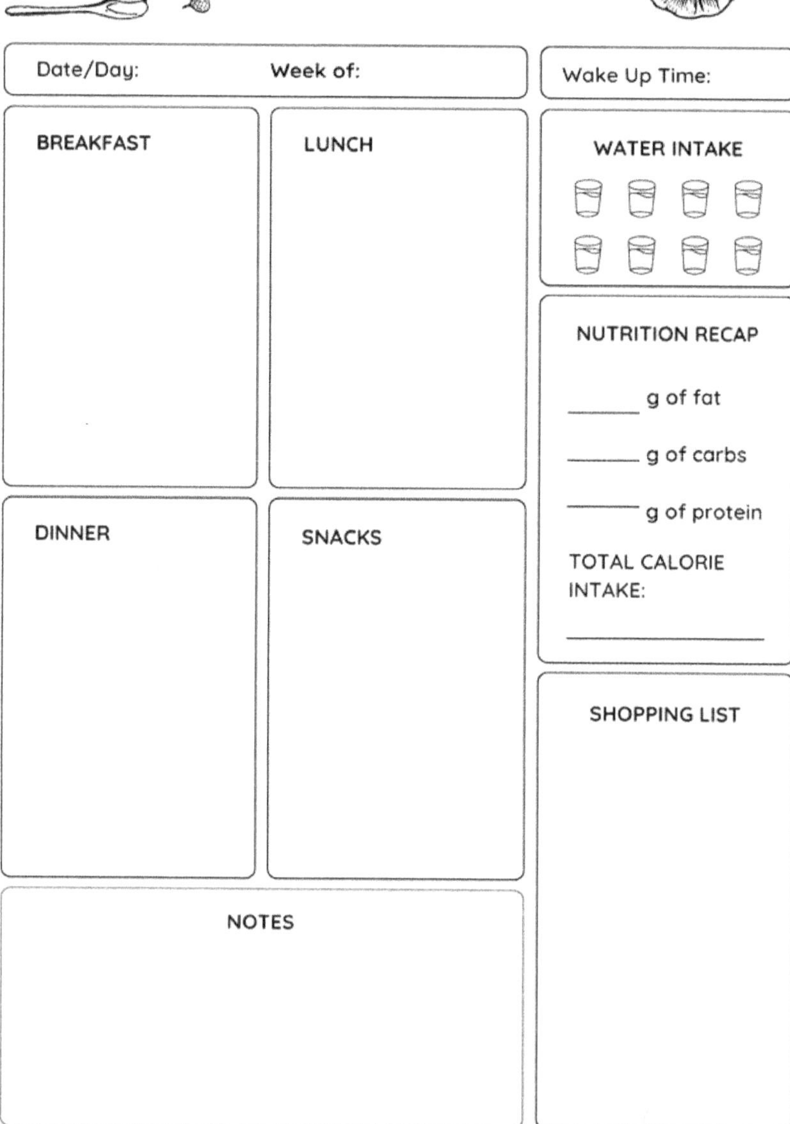

Date/Day: Week of:

Wake Up Time:

BREAKFAST

LUNCH

WATER INTAKE

DINNER

SNACKS

NUTRITION RECAP

_______ g of fat

_______ g of carbs

_______ g of protein

TOTAL CALORIE INTAKE:

____

SHOPPING LIST

NOTES

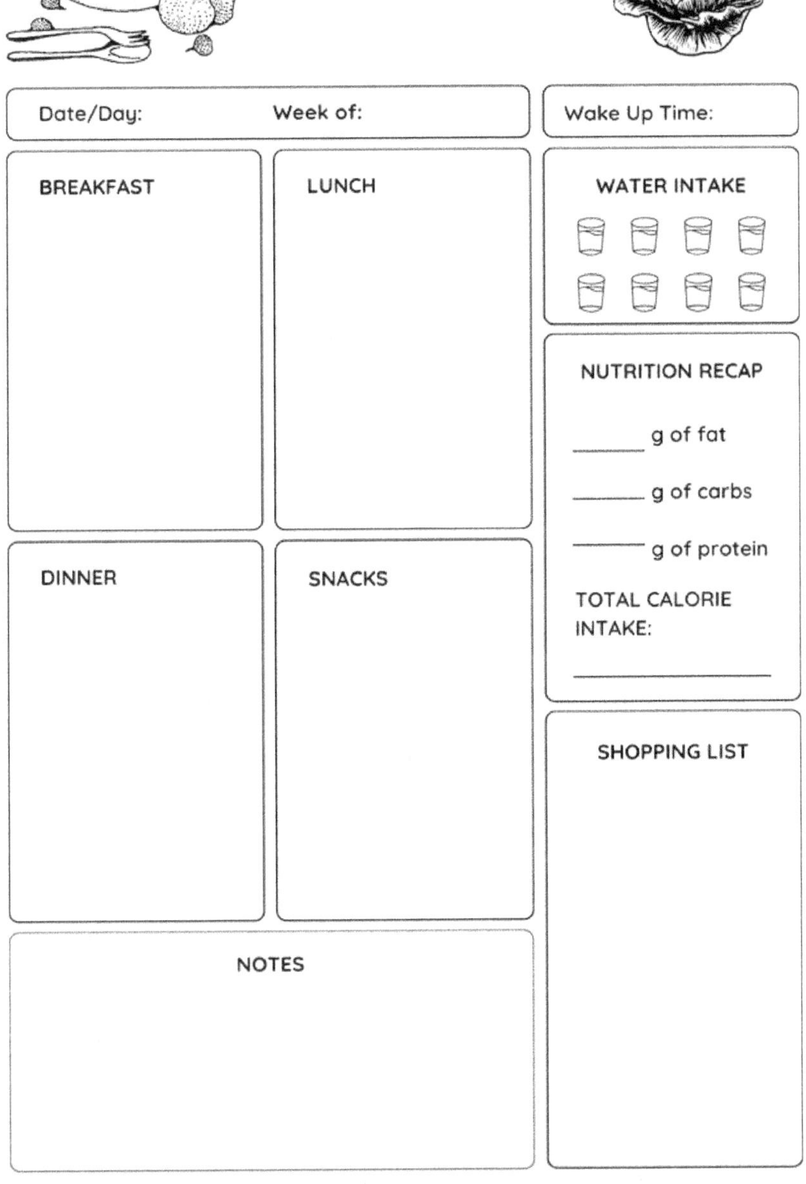

| Date/Day: | Week of: | Wake Up Time: |

BREAKFAST

LUNCH

WATER INTAKE

NUTRITION RECAP

_______ g of fat

_______ g of carbs

_______ g of protein

TOTAL CALORIE INTAKE:

____

DINNER

SNACKS

SHOPPING LIST

NOTES

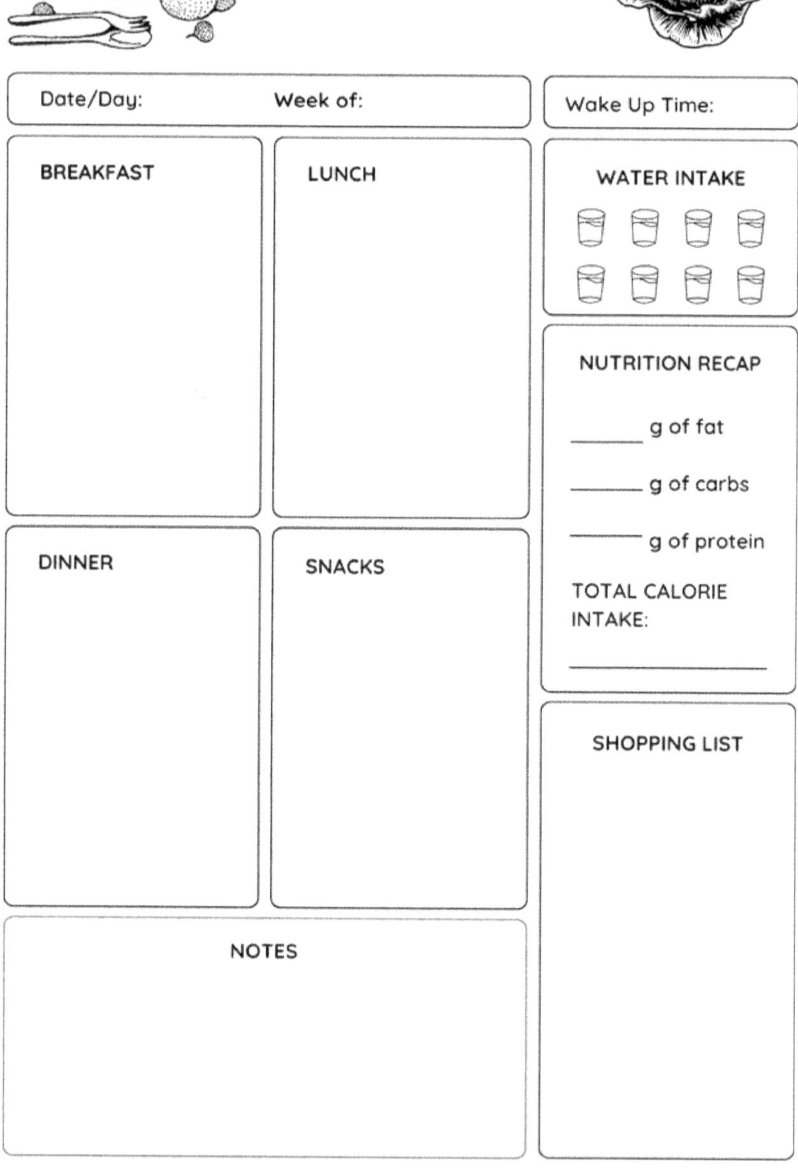

Date/Day:
Week of:
Wake Up Time:
BREAKFAST
LUNCH
WATER INTAKE
DINNER
SNACKS
NUTRITION RECAP
_______ g of fat
_______ g of carbs
_______ g of protein
TOTAL CALORIE INTAKE:
SHOPPING LIST
NOTES

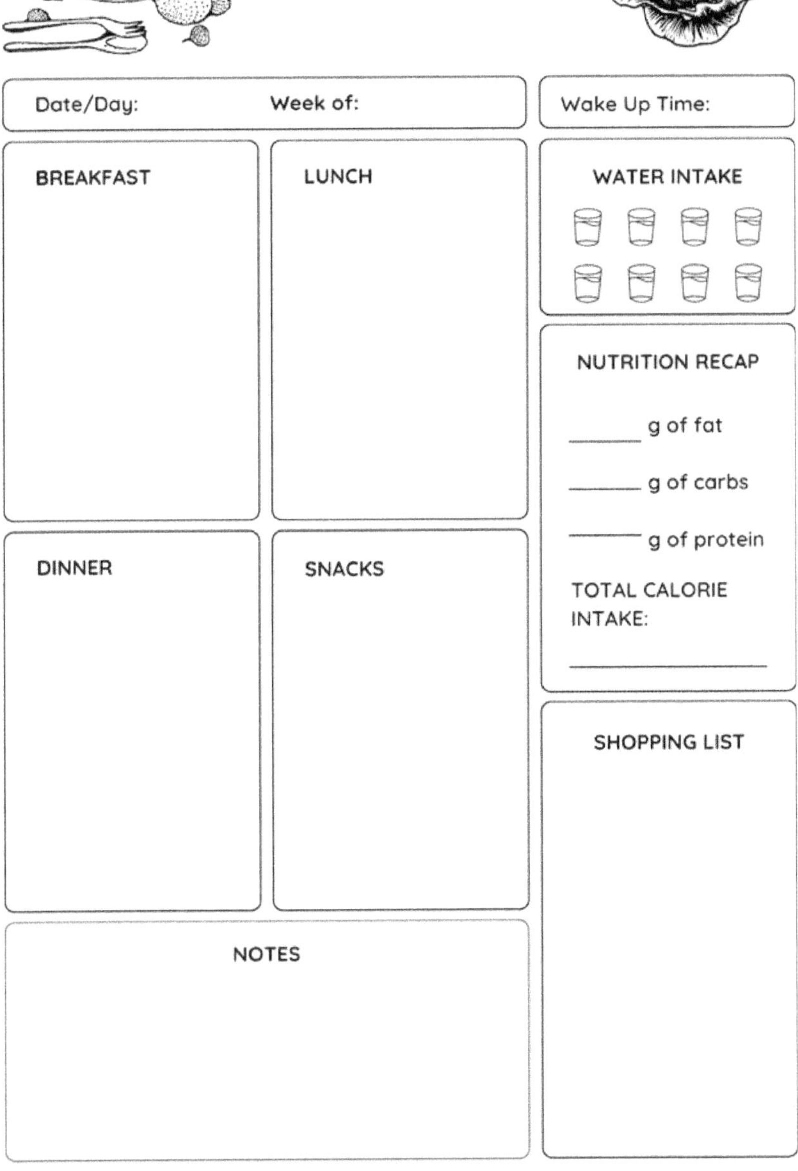

Date/Day:
Week of:
Wake Up Time:
BREAKFAST
LUNCH
WATER INTAKE
NUTRITION RECAP
_______ g of fat
_______ g of carbs
_______ g of protein
TOTAL CALORIE INTAKE:
DINNER
SNACKS
SHOPPING LIST
NOTES

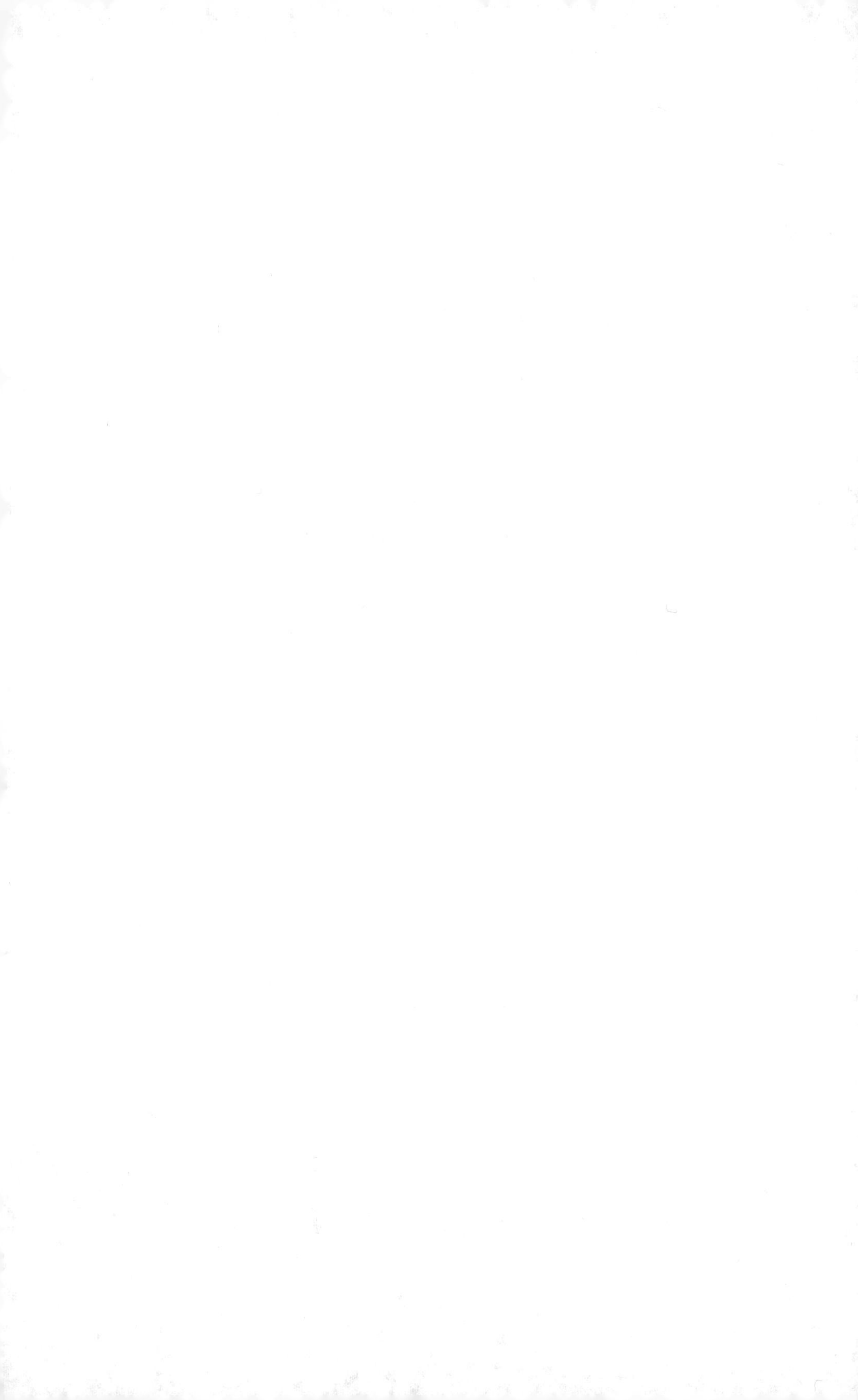

www.ingramcontent.com/pod-product-compliance
Lightning Source LLC
Chambersburg PA
CBHW072246260726
48659CB00004BA/1393